Rev[...]
Fami[...]

"Through her inspirin[...] [...]a Chaudhry interweaves hu[...] at engages anyone seeking to find balance through [...] [...]ny trials. This memorable work is an emotional and intellectual journey of how pain and suffering can coexist with love and hope. Reading this honest and poignant memoir, we are quickly reminded about the importance of valuing loved ones while they're still with us and cherishing every moment. Chaudhry's personal narrative strikes a chord, prompting us as readers to engage in vital conversations about our organ donation choices with those we hold dear. I highly recommend this book to anyone looking for an inspiring read that leaves a long-lasting impact."

SIMONNE WEEKS
Director of University of Brighton's Donor Research Group

~

"Family Matters is a very touching and beautifully written real-life story underlining the importance of organ donation and the need for more donors especially from various ethnic groups. I hope it inspires people to consider themselves as donors to give the Gift of Life as organ transplantation is life-saving and life-changing."

FRANK J.M.F. DOR
Consultant Transplant Surgeon

~

"Thank you, Aisha, for writing up this informative and thought-provoking life journey. Your mom's life was beautifully described in the book and reminded us all that transplantation is the gold standard treatment of choice for patients with organ failure. The success of human organ transplantation relies on the willingness of the public to donate their organs, either during their lifetime or after death. Regrettably, ethnic minorities, particularly the South Asian community, continue to exhibit low organ donation rates, resulting in a disproportionate number of South Asians waiting for transplants due to the frequent finding of suitable matches among members of the same ethnic group. This results in a disproportionate number of Asians waiting longer for transplants than the average waiting time. Sadly, many who are waiting count down their days on the list and lead an agonising life due to the scarcity of matching organ donors. How to raise awareness among South Asians about the scarcity of organ donors is a growing challenge for the UK and global health care systems. I truly hope that, through your book, many of your readers will acknowledge the need to register as potential organ donors and be the messengers of the "Gift of Life" message. Lack of knowledge about the need for organ donation is one of the major obstacles we are facing as a community, and we all have a role to play in raising awareness about this important topic. Over a decade of my voluntary work promoting organ and stem cell donors from the Asian community has been really rewarding. Thank you for all you do to help others and promote the *"Gift of Life"* message."

DR. AGIMOL PRADEEP BEM RN PNA
Senior Transplant coordinator & BAME Organ and Stem Cell Donor Campaigner"

~

I laughed and cried with equal intensity when I read this book. Aisha paints a vivid picture of happy memories, family ties and love, set against the backdrop of pain and frustration relating to the need for a donated kidney to save her mother's life, and the complexities of raising this as a conversation within her community. Her writing style enables the emotions she discusses, to leap from the words and straight into your heart and leaves you with an understanding of the importance of organ donation, and its huge impact on people's lives."

KATIE DOMBROWE
Paediatric Palliative Care Nurse

~

"A heartfelt emotional rollercoaster charting the journey of life. Organ failure does not discriminate and impacts upon families from different socio-economic, ethnic, and faith backgrounds. Family Matters shows that there is still so much for us to do in terms of normalising conversations about organ donation and end of life care. This endeavour is not an easy one and requires collective action at all levels of society – schools, colleges, universities, employers, media, politicians, celebrities, etc. – where organ donation should be routinely discussed, and visibility of the stories of living donors and donor families of deceased donors becomes the norm. Aisha and her family embarked on an incredible journey to save their mother, but their journey continues to save other people's lives, and it is our collective societal responsibility to provide companionship on this journey."

GURCH RANDHAWA PHD FFPH DL
Professor of Diversity in Public Health & Institute for Health Research, University of Bedfordshire

~

"Having worked in the scientific solid organ transplant area for so long I seemed to know most aspects in this area. When I read this book however it struck me with its heartbreaking and so personal emotional story. There are so many objective rational non-emotional fact driven stories/reports that it is fantastic to find an emotional appeal which tells the story of the life's journey that shows that such a tragic fate can happen to everyone and that the victims can as well be everyone - so no one must feel safe no matter how well they are and strong they may feel."

DR. SAMSON FUNG, M.D.
Fung Consulting

~

"Aisha effortlessly takes the reader through her family's journey of immigration, cultural integration, and everyday life around this. There are so many layers to unpack that speak to love, courage, hope, and loss. Inherently, the message is a call to action for health equity, raising awareness of organ donation and the difference that 'a gift of life' can make in communities most disadvantaged in access to transplantation. However, as each chapter unfolds, Aisha brings attention to wider issues related to equality and justice in society. Reading this book as an academic, a mother, and a daughter, I am encouraged that it will serve as a reminder that we all have power to think and do differently."

SHIVANI SHARMA
Professor of Health Equity and Inclusion, Aston University, Birmingham, UK

~

"Organ donation saves lives and can give hope to another in need but is still a taboo in many ethnic communities. Family Matters is beautifully written, a deeply affecting story. Packed with fun, love, family bonding and emotions, Aisha's narrative is both sensitive and incisive, deftly handling topics we often avoid. This memoir clearly put the spotlight on the reasons behind a lack of organ donors among non-white communities, which is a real eye opener. Aisha's message is very clear to everyone; register your decision to donate, and very importantly, discuss your wishes with your family. This is an essential read for all those interested in organ donation".

NELSON SELVARAKJ
Lecturer (Adult Nursing) at Cardiff University / Prifysgol

~

"The bitter truth is that most patients on the organ transplant waiting list from South Asian communities will die waiting due to the dearth of donated organs from members of these communities. This bitterly honest, viscerally raw, emotionally charged memoir is the campaign of one bereaved daughter who has lost her mother in her 10-year fight to find a life-saving kidney. Chaudhry marshals all her literary and practical skills with deft and dexterity to conjure up for us an image of the emotional roller coaster and tumultuous journey her whole family experienced preceding her mother's death. This memoir comes from a place of care; that no one should go through what she, her mother and her family went through. It is a heartfelt plea to South Asian communities to understand the importance of organ donation."

DR MANSUR ALI
Senior Lecturer in Islamic Studies, Cardiff University, UK.

~

"Aisha's 'Family Matters' is a very heartwarming read. In this memoir, she takes us through the heart- wrenching experience of the frustrations, trials and tribulations faced by her wonderful family, losing their precious mum who spent years waiting for a kidney transplant. The book raises the importance of all of us having that conversation with our loved ones about our wishes to donate organs. The statistics provided are eye opening and shows how urgent a topic this is, to save lives and improve the quality of many more lives. With her style of writing, Aisha engages with the reader really well. Highly recommended."

BINDHU XAVIER
Research Nurse

~

"Aisha's book is a beautiful testimonial and tribute to her mother. It shares the emotional gravity of love, and the experience of loss, and where love continues while feeling loss over the years. It is also a door that opens for others to recognize the why behind loving people's passions to build something beautiful for others, and I find Aisha's painstaking efforts to make known organ donation and its life-changing importance heroic. By using her words, she places a true cape by way of her book to fly into the hands of millions to read and feel the experience, so their decisions for their own lives can be the ones who save others as well. It's quite poetic. It's also impactful. We can clearly see what her superpower is here, through her origin story, and I look forward to see her words impact the world, generations unlimited."

ANITA MYERS
Life and Relationship Coach

~

"Aisha's story is so important oso many levels. It depicts the lives of a loving family through the normal challenges of life, as well as the stress of illness and the grief of loss. It demonstrates the importance of families having the important conversation about organ donation, especially those with Asian heritage because there are currently less opportunities for them to receive a lifesaving transplant. I hope this poignant story will encourage people to think about and discuss organ donation with their loved ones."

KAREN ROCKELL- *Patient Co-Director, Liver Transplant Recipient and Co-Director UK Organ Donation and Transplantation Research Network*

~

"This book provides a glimpse into Aisha's life, her experiences and strong family relationships. The essence of the Asian community its values, united strength in times of adversity are depicted beautifully. Extremely relatable to me both in terms of family, culture and organ donation."

MINI KARUPPAN
Organ Transplant Recipient

~

Family Matters
A Memoir

How living with hope despite
inevitable loss makes you stronger

AISHA CHAUDHRY

LLB (Hons), PG DIP Law, Certified Coach and NLP
Practitioner, Accredited Geographer of Emotions

For every purchase of this memoir a small donation
of money or books will be made to an organisation or
charity working on improving patient's lives who are
waiting for an organ donation.

Copyright ©Aisha Chaudhry, 2024

Cover illustration: Petra Wendler
Second paperback print edition: 2024

www.happyaisha.com
email: familymattersbook@hotmail.com

The right of Aisha Chaudhry to be identified
as the author of this book has been asserted.

ISBN 978-3-9826288-1-3

For Daddy Ajaz

You took on the role of Mum and Daddy and you did a great job. You let me into your life and I let you into mine.

This book is about my mum who was waiting for a kidney transplant and lost her fight for life. My aim is to raise awareness about organ donation

Aisha Chaudhry

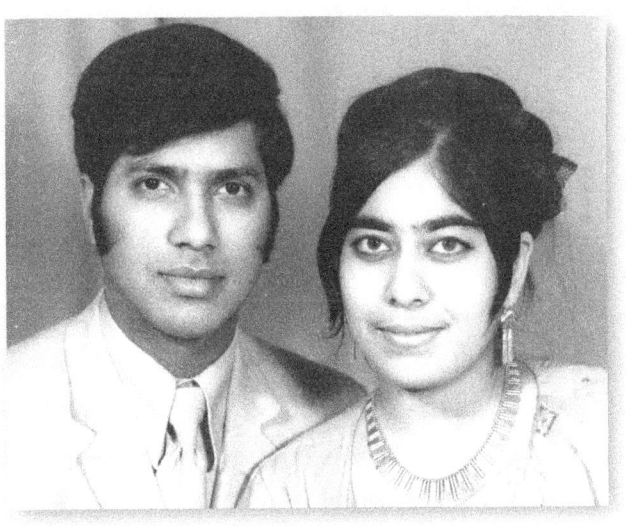

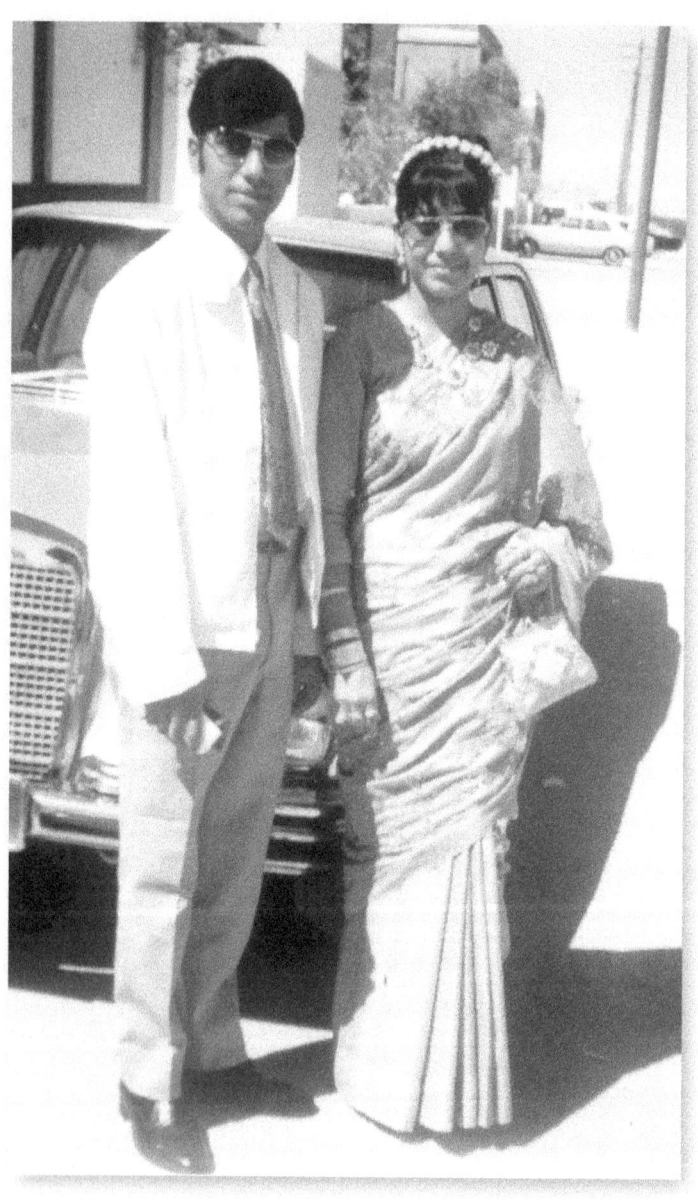

Prologue

I was raised in a household where young girls were treated the same way as their brothers. This is because I grew up with a strong-willed mother who wanted all four of us children to be equally independent. Mum's attitude toward life set me up with the right mindset about how to be respectful, and kind, but also how to be firm. I knew what to expect as a woman in life. I have my mother's character as a courageous fighter (despite her waiting in vain for an organ transplant) to thank for that.

Why I Resumed Writing this Memoir

I gave each of my family members a hug. I stood back saying out loud how I wondered if this would be the last time that we would see each other for a while because of this pandemic. It seemed to be killing people from all over the world; nobody knew enough about it. As I stepped back, I cried. I was looking at my family thinking, *Will I see you again, or will this virus kill all of us?*

It was 16 March 2020, as I walked through London Heathrow Airport to my departure gate. Everyone was required to wear masks to protect themselves and others from this unknown virus. Wearing a mask felt not only unfamiliar but odd. I boarded the flight back to Berlin from the UK. I took a photo from my seat of the beautiful crimson sky as the sun was setting. My mouth was covered with what felt like a cardboard mask that we had all been instructed to wear, because nobody knew much about the coronavirus at the time. I struggled to focus through the constant build-up of steam on my glasses.

I felt uncomfortable, even unsettled. I had knots in my stomach that were familiar to me, but not in the good way. The departure triggered a huge wave of emotions inside of me that mirrored those from when my mother passed away in 2001. I felt nauseous and dizzy. My mouth was dry. I felt shivery, and my legs were shaking involuntarily.

I had this feeling deep in my gut that things were going to get difficult and bad once again. Last time it was my family who was suffering; this time the whole world. Everything was out of our control; like it had been when Mum was unwell. This feeling of fear, of unknown territory, was right back there again in the pit of my stomach. I felt a lump form in my throat. I realised on that aeroplane, as I looked out to the earth below, which was so far away from the sky above, that I was thinking a lot about my Mum. What would she have made of it all? It dawned on me again how young Mum was when she died, since she had only just turned fifty years old.

People didn't seem to die from old age anymore. In fact, this virus was showing the world that you could die at any age. Over the coming year, the media reported an enormous number of deaths, showing plenty of disturbing video footage.

I watched as coffins piled up in the Italian province of Bergamo as Italians struggled to bury their dead. People in Pakistan couldn't get enough oxygen to support their breathing. There were bodies on the streets in Ecuador that had nowhere to be placed. India held mass outdoor cremations during which the heat from the fires looked unbearable. At home, I sat wondering if life would ever be the same again.

It reminded me of a deep sadness. Watching Mum die was heart-breaking, but I was there with her. I felt privileged that I had managed to be so close to her when she was dying. She wasn't alone. Twenty years later, I was watching families being ripped away from their sick loved ones forever, forbidden from being allowed to go near them. People wearing hazmat suits in hospitals were trying to help so many patients, many of whom had died alone.

It was March 2001 when I first started to write down my thoughts, which eventually became this memoir. It was March 2020 when I found myself opening my memoir to continue writing. I wanted to record my emotions through my memories - an urge I hadn't felt since after my Mum died. It was a way to process my feelings, acknowledging to myself that no one knows when they will die. If I wanted to share my story – aged forty-five at the time of writing – only five years away from the age Mum was when she died, then I needed not to wait. The future wasn't that clear for anyone anymore, so I had to get on with it now.

I knew I had an incredibly important message to pass on to the world. I hoped it would prevent other daughters or sons from experiencing the same sort of loss that I had. My Mum died on 3 February 2001, after waiting for a kidney transplant for ten years. She had been cared for by the amazing staff at the Royal Berkshire Hospital in Reading, Berkshire, where she had dialysis every other day. Being able to dialyse is what kept her alive, and we were all grateful for that. I had lived life throughout the ten years from 1991 until 2001, while she was a kidney transplant patient, fully hoping that she would get a telephone call saying a kidney had been found for her. I truly believed that.

A kidney dialysis machine does the job of the kidneys for as long as your body can take it. It can be draining on the body. The process involves the removal of the waste and excess fluid from the blood that your kidneys are no longer able to filter out. There are two types of dialysis: Haemodialysis (HD) which filters your blood using a machine and a synthetic membrane, called a dialyser. HD is performed in a hospital or dialysis center. It can also be performed at home. Peritoneal dialysis (PD) uses dialysis fluid and the lining of your abdomen, called the peritoneal membrane, to filter your blood inside your body. PD can be performed in your own home daily[1].

Your quality of life is compromised because you don't have the freedom of time you were once used to having. If you are on dialysis[2], your time is restricted, as is your ability to walk freely since you are connected by tubes to a rather large machine. It's not something that can be carried around. An organ transplant, on the other hand, isn't a cure, but keeps you mostly out of the hospital, opening up the chance for you to live a better quality of life with your family. That's what my siblings and I had all hoped for throughout the ten years that my mother spent waiting.

That time in my life was turbulent because we were living on edge, not knowing which way things would turn whenever Mum got an infection. It often resulted in her having to stay in the hospital.

Being so clearly focused on living her best life with her family, she rarely spoke to us about her thoughts or feelings deep inside. She didn't want us to worry more than we already did. We knew not to ask too many questions and could see her suffering with our own eyes. I am sure she spoke about how she really felt in confidence to her four best friends who were adults. I felt reassured that she had such friendships with these other caring Asian women in the community.

I think not complaining had to do with her dignity and humility. She didn't need the whole community to know everything she was feeling, which was possibly because she wanted people to remember her as a normal person in the Asian community who was simply making the best out of their situation. I think she also believed that it didn't help to verbalise the difficulties of life on dialysis and the impact it had on her body. Most times it went well; it was keeping her alive after all. Instead she preferred to focus living life as best as she could. It meant people believed she would eventually get better. Unfortunately, it didn't work that way.

When my mother passed away, I was angry to my core. She had actually finally died. What we only ever imagined would happen late in our parents lives, had become reality for us, only much earlier than expected. Our parents were meant to live long lives before dying, but for Mum, her life had been stripped away far too soon.

Having turned from forty-nine to fifty years of age, literally five days after her birthday she had been admitted to hospital; but this time she didn't make it home. Little did I know that her journey in life on a kidney dialysis machine would be for as long as it was, or that her life span would be so drastically shortened. A truly tragic dichotomy. She had missed out on a long life with those who loved her as a daughter, a sister, a wife, a mother, a friend, and a grandmother to her grandchildren whom she never met.

Because Mum was of Asian heritage, getting a kidney was going to be harder since there simply weren't enough Asian people in the UK who had volunteered, in the case of their own deaths, to donate a kidney to save another life. Unlike other organs, kidney donors need to be matched by blood group and tissue type. People from the same ethnic background are more likely to be a match. Her chances of a match were much higher with a donor from a similar background. I do not want another family, especially a Black, Asian, or East Asian family, to suffer what I suffered. Even one person and their family, who suffers like mine did, is one family too many.

There have been extraordinary medical advances in life-changing donations by now. Donation registers range from blood, platelet, plasma, bone marrow, and tissue to cord blood banks. Yet although the number of people waiting for a transplant has gone up, there are ironically still not enough organ donors.

A change in law[3] in all four countries of the United

Kingdom made it automatically the case that one would be on the organ donor register unless one opted out. This means within a soft opt-out system for organ donation (also known as presumed consent), everyone is considered to agree to donate their organs when they die unless they record a decision not to donate - (opting out) – or are in one of the excluded groups. Most importantly, this soft opt-out law means the wishes of the family members will be considered.

By October 2023, the latest "NHS Blood and Transplant Annual Report on Ethnicity Differences in Organ Donation and Transplantation"[4] showed that people from ethnic minorities are still significantly underrepresented in organ donation. A major problem is the decline in family consent or authorisation rates across all ethnic groups after a person has died.

Despite the change in the law, relatives will still be consulted first about whether organ donation is possible when there is no clear expression of the deceased's wishes. Relatives have been known to block the wishes of their family member who didn't express their decision to donate to their relatives[5]. It is therefore still extremely important to register your decision to donate and discuss it with your family so that they can have peace of mind knowing that your decision is being honoured.

In 2023, the number of potential ethnic minority donors in the UK was 750 (out of 600,000 deaths overall) and of that, only 246 were actual ethnic minority donors (Figure 1). In contrast, 1,106 transplant patients from ethnic minority groups received an organ with a further 2,237 patients from ethnic minority groups on the waiting list. Strikingly, 80% of transplants in people from ethnic minority groups were from white donors. Out of the 246 donations from patients in ethnic minority groups, 138 were from living donors. This means people from ethnic minority groups are more comfortable giving an organ while they are alive, but paradoxically families often decide against organ donation when a member is deceased.

Cultural beliefs about donation put families in a very awkward and difficult position because there is no worse time to seek consent on a tough decision than when family members are grieving the death of a loved one.

The main reasons families from ethnic minority backgrounds have in the past decided not to give consent or authorisation for organ donation of their deceased's organs, was due to it being against their religious and cultural beliefs (Table 1).

Other reasons were being unsure whether the patient would have agreed to donation or not knowing enough about it. Some families' decisions stemmed from stigmas against organ donation which have existed because of a mistrust in the healthcare system. The mistrust resulted from organ donor scandals at hospitals or from the market for trafficking organs for money. All of these obstacles meant the odds of Mum getting a suitable donor were stacked up against her – making it a predictable tragedy waiting to happen.

The number of deceased donors is still dire and way too low. At the same time, people from ethnic minority groups are overrepresented in the number of active opt-outs relative to the general population (Figure 2), leading altogether to the situation that people from ethnic minorities have to wait longer for an organ because the number of people waiting is greater.

This is not only a British but an international phenomenon. The Council of Europe Transplant Newsletter highlighted the total number of transplant rates in general, and kidney transplant rates in particular from deceased and living donors internationally.[6] Countries with predominantly non-white populations had incredibly low transplant numbers (Figures 3 and 4).[7]

I hope my experiences will encourage readers who have

intentionally opted out from the organ donor register to reconsider. If a person decides to opt back into the organ donor register because of reading my book, I will be thrilled. Together we could make all the difference in the lives of the many patients waiting.

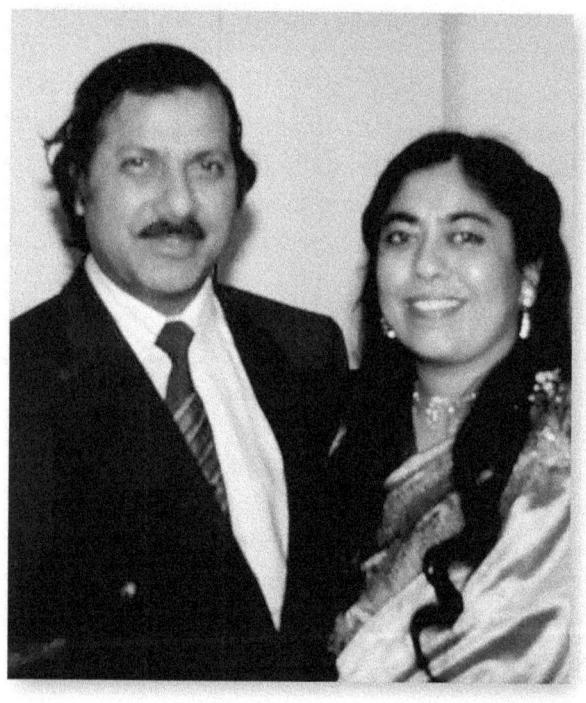

In Conclusion

The problem of a lack of organ donors among non-white communities has not been solved at all. Far from it. Only by speaking out and talking to our loved ones can we get this message heard.

I hope my story will encourage you to have that conversation about what your family member's wish is at the end of their lives. If they choose to be an organ donor, to give the gift of life to those patients waiting for a life-saving transplant, then it's important that the deceased's family know to give consent to the donation.

The topic of organ donation isn't comfortable to spring into, but I can tell you – and this memoir will show you – losing our loved ones when it could have been avoided hurts like hell. This brings me to the most important message: family matters. Ask yourself this:

- Would you take a human organ to survive or prolong your life?
- How many times have you watched or thought about someone you know who is suffering because of a health issue?
- What is the best thing that could happen when you agree to donate your organs?

My hope is that this memoir – written by a proud British Asian, born in Reading, Berkshire, England, now a proud German citizen – will prompt you to talk to your families about your organ donation intentions. You do not have to wait to talk about organ donation until it becomes that uncomfortable topic staring you in the face when death already is. At that crucial point, time is of the essence and is running out because organs need to be saved within hours of death. By then, emotions are high, thinking isn't clear, and for your loved one, the end is imminent.

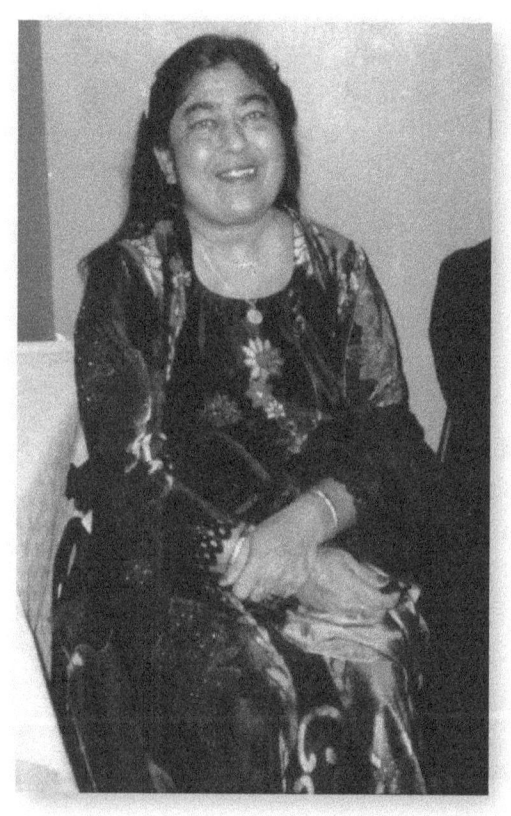

Chapter 1
A Sea of Sadness

Mum's Passing

None of us were at home in Reading when we headed to the intensive care unit in London to see what was happening with Mum. Ten years earlier, we were a normal Asian family of two hard-working parents and four kids, all getting on with our busy lives. Our parents did their best to give each of us a happy childhood. I felt safe knowing I was protected by them, which is what every kid should feel growing up. They were always there to watch over us whenever possible. I never ever felt like anything bad could happen to me as a child growing up with my parents and siblings. It could be because they kept an eye on us, letting us only participate in something if there was adult supervision. It's only now that I realise how they never argued in front of us; in fact, they never argued at all.

That meant my childhood was a harmonious one; or to put it another way, once we found out Mum was unwell, we had other worries on our minds. Difficult situations sometimes lead to families breaking apart. In other instances, it brings them closer together, making them stronger; like it had done with mine.

Here we were, ten years later, being told by the surgeon he was finally ready to operate on Mum's heart. Daddy, my youngest brother, my twin sister Aneesa, and myself had made it in time to see her shortly before she was taken in for surgery. Only my oldest brother Abbid didn't make it in time. Mum was in a critical condition where every minute counted, so they didn't wait.

The surgeon explained how he held her heart in his hands while he was trying to deal with the infection she had. He told us they resuscitated her three times while she lay on the operating table. Her life was *literally* in his hands. He said the operation was a success and that he was happy with his efforts. He seemed to be reassuring himself by saying, "I've done my part; now it's up to her." What I understood that to mean was him saying, "It's not on me if she doesn't have the strength to pull through."

It was up to her to show she wanted it enough - to live! Her willpower to live was so incredibly strong. Of course she wanted to live! Then he added, in the same sentence, that she only had a 25% chance of survival. We had to wait and see how things developed. Was she going to make it? For us, it was a waiting game.

She held on to life for over a week. She was fighting for her life, even managing to sing our younger brother Happy birthday. Then, in the second week, her signs of improvement slowed down. The night of February 2nd was an uncomfortably long night for all of us to get through, but each of us had hope. Hope was always there.

The following morning, we went to the intensive care unit but she wasn't in the open ward anymore. They had moved her to a room. Waiting for someone to tell us what was going on felt like an eternity. The consultant approached us slowly. I had a bad feeling in my gut. My emotions were running high, leaving me sweating profusely. Tears were welling up in my eyes as he said they couldn't offer her any more care. In fact, it was only a matter of time. She was dying. I processed what we had been told, feeling emotionally depleted of hope. I was so disappointed - gutted that they had given up on her.

It came as a complete shock; despite the warnings we had been given earlier. He said it wasn't clear how long it would take, but that we should spend the rest of the time with her. Then he told us which room she was in. Broken by the news, I stared at him, waiting for him to say something else. He didn't. He walked away. I froze with fear, literally unable to move, as I took in his words. Time stood still for a moment, leaving me feeling numb, but my thoughts were running fast through my head. I refused to believe it. I didn't want to accept it, but apparently it was true. The only way to check if he was right would be to see with my own eyes that he wasn't lying to us. Then I could be sure it wasn't a horrible mistake.

As we waited to go into the room, I slowly opened the door to peek. I could see the nurses were cleaning her up, because there was so much blood on her. One of the nurses suddenly looked up, pausing from her work. I had caught her eye. She looked irritated that I had seen the state of Mum before they were ready to let us in. It was like seeing a painting that still needed the final touches before a public viewing. I closed the door gently, waiting until we finally got invited into her room. A few minutes later, we were led in by a nurse who looked solemnly at us. We walked in one by one, surrounding her. Daddy was closest to her. It was eerily quiet and incredibly uncomfortable. Mum had lost her lease for life, all because she didn't get the kidney transplant she desperately needed. Her body had gone through ten years of dialysis along with multiple infections. Her heart couldn't take any more. It was giving up. She was still alive, but we were losing her. She was losing us. I felt sorry that Mum's life was going to end this way, but nothing more could have been done to save her.

The beeping sound from the machines rang loud in my ears. The tubes were still attached. I can still visualise everything, even now. The colour of the blanket was slightly off white, while the machines were a pale blue. The oxygen tubes were clear, while the other tubes were red from blood. The lines on the screen had different colours. The monitor showed her vital signs. The line of her heartbeat was moving slowly. It was all there to see. Nothing had been switched off, thank goodness. For that short moment, time stood still, just like we did, not saying anything. I looked at Mum, wondering what she must have been feeling. I imagine she would have been scared, heartbroken and devastated at what was happening to her; that she had lost her family who meant so much to her. She had lost her fight to live her life.

One nurse said that twelve units of blood had been given to her to keep her alive. You do that when you are trying to save a life. The nurses must have been doing their best to keep her alive, right? My head was pounding hard. I was scared, wondering if she would somehow miraculously make it. That was me giving myself false hope. Then, one nurse asked in a gentle voice if we still wanted her to receive blood since it wouldn't keep her alive but would slow down her death. She wasn't going to benefit from it because she was now dying.

I felt a punch in my stomach, knowing they were asking us indirectly if the blood could be saved for someone else who might live from receiving it versus giving it to Mum who was going to die. They waited for our answer. My stomach turned. What should we say? I could see creases on our foreheads from the strain we were feeling from the question we had sensitively been asked.

We all seemed to agree collectively to stop giving her more blood. Now they could give it to someone else who was going to benefit from it. Thinking about it, I realise how much they did to try to keep her alive; they resuscitated her several times on the operating table; they gave her twelve units of blood. They kept her connected to all the machines right until the end.

Mum had a small tear in her eye. It was the last tear she would ever shed. I stared fixating my own eyes on it. I held her soft, frail hand. It was a light, pale colour.

Each tear that hit the back of my throat as I swallowed left a sweet taste at the back of my aching throat. How it ached. It was unbearable. We didn't know how long it would take. Nor could we truly believe what was happening. All the tissues I had on me were soaked from my tears. My eyebrows were frowning tightly together. While my lips were pursed shut, I found myself gritting my teeth whilst trying to comprehend what I was seeing. I felt waves of sadness gushing through my entire body while letting out heavy sighs of air through my mouth. I could feel my heart race faster, then it calmed down for a few moments only to race faster again.

We tried to keep it together for Daddy too because we realised how difficult this was for him, but it was impossible. He was understandably emotional during that time, holding Mum's hand. We saw a vulnerable side of him. We were all in the moment together entranced by how still Mum was lying there, and the fast speed at which the day passed.

The next eleven hours saw each of us witness how Daddy was collecting his thoughts, but not speaking much. We dipped in and out of conversation with him, all the while being extremely aware of how hard it must have been for him to see his life partner dying in front of his eyes. None of us were distracted by anything outside of room seven. Daddy hugged his children so much that day. He was fragile, like an eggshell that was barely intact.

All our hearts were broken. Our hope, gone. It had been replaced with despair. I was looking at Mum on the bed, lying still. I kept turning my head towards the machine half expecting it to surprise us with some miracle. All of this was going on while we were waiting for a signal from the nurses that there had been a mistake, that she would live after all. Hope had been by my side all along, but now it was teasing me. The sound of the machines seemed to get louder, as did we from all of us crying. The noise coming from the machines was like an orchestra playing a cacophony of discordant sounds.

They were deafening despite the quietness in the room. My sensitivity was heightened because I felt fragile and wounded; broken and sad. I was confused because the sounds from the machines were steadily leading me to think nothing bad was going to happen. I even convinced myself for a short time that it meant Mum was still going to live. I believed Mum could hear us all the time. She was crying with her family too. From around 10:00 am that day, we each sat with her, stroking her face gently, holding her soft, frail, pale hands. I told her all of the thoughts that came into my head, whispering them into her ear. I told her how I didn't want her to go; how I wanted to learn to cook better; how I was probably going to live and work abroad for a bit; how I didn't know what would happen to Daddy without her; how I needed her to tell me what to expect from life as a woman; how I would do my best to look out for each of us children, and how I would keep an eye on Daddy. I know she heard me loud and clear because they say hearing is the last thing to go.

Then, at 1:30 pm, we were thrown out of our fixation on Mum when one of the nurses said it was starting to happen. She was dying. We didn't know how long it would take, but we could see her heartbeat rhythm on the monitor right up until it began to slow down. I know the exact time. I know the exact point – Annsa's heartbeat line went flat on the screen. It was like what you see in the movies. Time stood still on the outside. The numbers on the machine had gone down to almost zero.

We were in a collective trance of togetherness. It slowly dawned on me that we would never be a family of six again. I never had an inkling that this would actually happen someday, but how it crept up on me suddenly was quite unexpected. I simply wasn't ready for it. I almost lost my balance while I stood with one foot on top of the other by Mum's bed, registering that thought. I wanted all of our family to be together for every single precious minute that passed, before moving on with life, like time already had. Paralysis gnawed at me, taking over, leaving me feeling sick, crushed, raw, and fragile. At the same time, there was an incredible feeling of love in the room.

The love we felt for Mum and for each other showed me what a strong bond our family had. We hugged and held hands surrounding Mum the entire time so she could feel it too. I am sure she could.

I took a moment to appreciate the enormity of what was happening. That experience felt like a ship that had cast its anchor forever into the deep blue sea, never to sail again. The sea was a flood of our tears. The tears created heavy waves across deep waters far away from what the naked eye could see. The ship was slowly sinking to the bottom because our world as we knew it had completely and utterly collapsed.

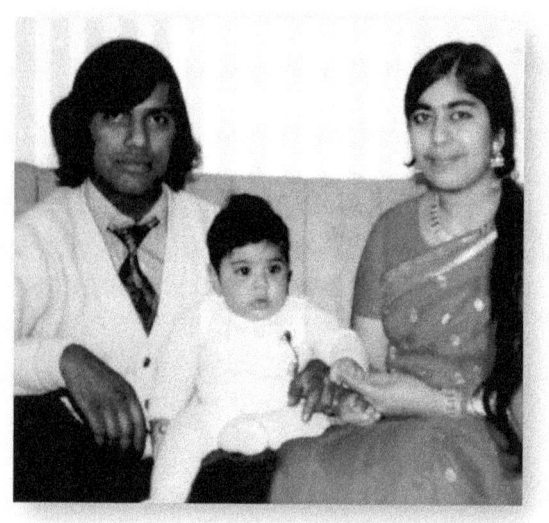

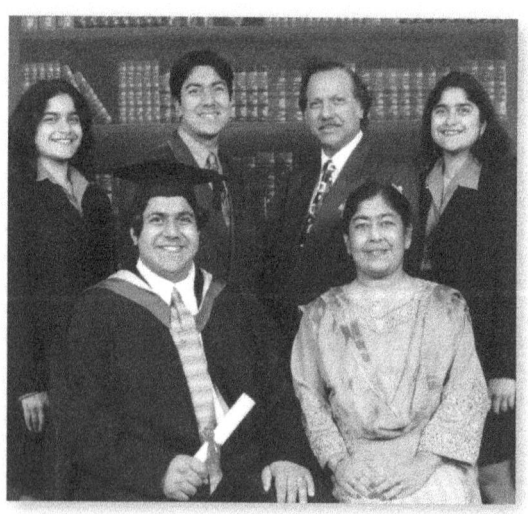

Chapter 2
Our Early Years, 1980

The Naughty Years

Often, after a long difficult day, Mum would come home feeling exhausted. One can imagine that giving birth to twins was difficult, but her two were a real pain. As if the fact of being pregnant wasn't trouble enough, Mum had to keep horizontal during her pregnancy for quite a few months to make sure we stayed safe inside her womb. We deceptively cute brown girls were a hyperactive, over-energetic pair, who would have been particularly exhausting for any parent.

I must admit that the fearsome thought of having to look after a pair of girls like us only compounds my respect for my Mum. When I got a bit older, I often asked Mum if we were worth it. After all, she had spent five months in the hospital bed hallucinating from medication while being unable to stand up in case we fell out. It was not an easy pregnancy, to say the least.

"Were we worth it, Mum?"

"Yes, of course, you were," she would say, smiling gently with real love shining out from her beautiful brown eyes. She smiled with her eyes.

I wouldn't say Aneesa and I were an ordinary pair of twins, but then, what is ordinary when you are a twin? I knew we weren't ordinary kids. Since the start, we have been nothing short of extraordinary. It was always so easy to feel special because as identical twins people noticed us. They stared at us for being dressed identically; for sounding exactly the same. We behaved similarly and spoke at double the speed of most kids our age. We finished off each other's sentences all the time. We were usually wide awake at 4 am, ready to play and have fun, and to conquer our little world. We were happy go lucky energetic kids.

"Different" is another suitable description of us. We really were double trouble, erring on the side of naughty. Actually, very naughty. You'd think that one of us would be the sensible one, holding the other back from our cheeky shenanigans, but nope, we would happily egg each other on. The more we talked, the more energy we got. We were running around like fully charged batteries letting out all of our energy so everyone around us could get some too. Of course, it also meant playing in the garden with each other, and tiring ourselves out so that Daddy would have to carry us upstairs to the bed after falling asleep on his or Mum's lap.

At the pioneering age of five, while on a breath-taking mission to climb the Himalayas, we had managed to climb up to the top of our own imaginary mountain. To a young child, this meant climbing up to the bathroom cabinet, which was located directly above the sink. We knew this was a no-go zone – the area at home you are forbidden to go to on your own. Did that stop us? Of course it didn't! Here was an opportunity for fun and adventure, which meant no rules applied. At least that's how we saw it. We had managed to manoeuvre up towards the bathroom cabinet, but how we did it remains a mystery to this day.

With one foot on the edge of the green bathroom sink, the other on the tip of the radiator, I forced open the door of the medicine cabinet while leaning the other hand against the wall, making sure not to fall. I could see the reflection of my face on the doors of the mirror. I peeked inside the cabinet. In front of me were some shiny, metal, rectangular-shaped objects stacked away on the top shelf that caught my attention. We knew what we were doing was naughty, but more importantly, it was fun.

Tucked away in a plastic cover was a packet of what I now know were double-sided single-use razor blades. The images of our faces squashed onto a tiny reflection from the sharp, searing razor blades seemed funny at the time. With big smiles on our faces, we felt rather proud of our discovery. Our parents, however, were horrified to see blood from the cuts that we had made all over our little hands, leaving a trail of tiny red handprints all over the white bathroom walls. Mischievous is what we were, and mischievous is what we still are, especially when there is fun to be had.

Even though we twins are grown-up adults now, we kept this spark of energy - a cheekiness deep inside us. Our bond as twins is definitely special. We could read each other's minds and finish off each other's sentences easily. We stuck up for the other whenever one of us needed defending. Because of the mighty force of nature that we were, neither Mum nor Daddy nor any of our teachers stood a chance at stamping this out of us. It's still there. Perhaps with the seriousness of life, all that has really changed are our lived experiences.

These incidents showed Mum at an early age how Aneesa and I had a huge amount of energy and curiosity. We were a strong pair of girls who operated as a rather sophisticated toddler unit. We certainly gave her and Daddy a lot to handle. Over time, our escapades landed us in trouble because of what we got up to. Mum saw quickly how we got a kick out of exploring whatever surrounded us. We constantly bounced off each other's energy. When she wasn't keeping an eye on us, we were always conjuring up something to have fun. In fact, once, we had taken all the wet clothes out of the washing machine and laid them out all across the floor. Because we did it together, we were really efficient.

We were mostly left to play together, only being interrupted when we were doing something naughty, which turned out to be quite a lot. Over the years, we learned to have fun, there were definitely boundaries about where we could go on our own, and how far from home. We were basically only allowed out of the front door and up and down the same road which made me feel like we had to earn the privilege to go outside. Needless to say, it wasn't very often and if we did go, it was with our older brother.

We presented Mum with so many challenges on a daily basis, that she usually knew when we were up to mischief. It usually started with us chatting loudly and then suddenly going quiet if something happened that was most likely to get us told off. It then followed with Mum telling us to come downstairs so she could check up on us and find out what we were getting up to. I guess it also showed her that we had each other's backs. We still look out for each other today. She's just not there to see it.

Emigrating from Pakistan

I have strong memories from when I was around seven-years-old of Daddy coming home from work. We greeted him with a glass of water or juice whenever he arrived through the door. Sometimes, he would relax in his armchair telling us stories from when he was a young boy before he moved to the United Kingdom. We listened to him while perching on either side of the armrests of the sofa. He talked about his parents, explaining in detail how his family had emigrated to the UK in the 1950s. Daddy was born in South Asia, in India, in a region which later in 1947 became Pakistan.

He re-told us stories of how, up until 1947, Pakistan had been taken over by the British Indian Empire, which ruled it until it had gained its independence. When I asked how he ended up emigrating from Pakistan to the UK, he explained it in his calm, soft voice. I could feel the deep sound of his voice echo through his entire chest cavity, while I leaned on it, listening. I loved leaning on his chest because it always felt safe. I used to compare that sound to when I held my violin under my chin whilst playing long low notes across the strings with my bow. The sound vibrated through the entire instrument just like Daddy's soft, deep voice would.

He described how in 1947, when he was two years old, the United Kingdom had agreed to the partitioning of India into three parts: India, Pakistan, and East Pakistan (now Bangladesh). During this time, there was also mass migration of Muslims, Hindus, and Sikhs.

Due to the increased tension resulting from the partition, lots of people lost their lives. Daddy went on to tell us how his father, Mohammad Shaffi Chaudhry, known to us grandchildren as Dadajaan, was born in 1912 in India. His job was working for the Regiment, which was part of the British Empire. Eventually, Dadajaan opened his own tailor business, where he made suits that were made to measure. He went from Lahore, where the family was living, to work in Karachi, Pakistan's capital at the time, so that he could expand his business to international tailoring. He knew a Sikh gentleman who encouraged him to emigrate with his family to England. The Sikh gentleman kept in touch with him, advising him to look at the future of his family, saying that if he wanted any guidance on emigrating abroad to the United Kingdom, he would happily help.

Pakistan had been newly created. Some people woke up to find India, their home country, had been split into three separate countries, leaving them with little idea of what to expect from all of the uncertainty. Having lived in India under British rule, the idea of moving to the United Kingdom seemed like a choice between familiarity versus the unknown. It was an option worth considering. With that in mind, Dadajaan went to the United Kingdom in 1954 on his own to explore prospects for a new future for his family. He went to a tailor and cutters hub on Gerrard Street, London, to become a certified tailor. This didn't take him long since he was able to demonstrate his skills easily. Within two years, he sold his business in Karachi, Pakistan, emigrating with his family to the UK.

During the time Dadajaan was working away in the UK, his family moved from a place called Model Town on the outskirts of Lahore, which was in the province of Punjab, to the province of Sindh, Karachi, where one of his sisters lived. From 1953 to 1956, Daddy went to a private English school. His headteacher, a British school teacher, would arrive at the school in a Rolls Royce car with her eight dogs. I wonder if that's why Daddy would stop us in the street whenever he saw a Rolls Royce, often admiring the vehicle.

Mum and Daddy's families knew each other from the time they lived in Karachi because one of his aunties had a great friendship with Mum's family. They used to go to his auntie's house for Mathematics and English tutoring. That house in Karachi was next door to the house where my Mum, Annsa Sabiha Noor lived when she was between three and five years old. It could be that my parents played on the same roof terraces on the top of the houses, maybe even at the same time. I guess we will never know.

When Mum was little, her parents separated which means she had two dads, both of whom she said she loved very much. She called one her father and the other one Daddy. I thought this was cool. She spent time growing up around them both. She told us often that she loved both families very much.

After the partition, in the shadow of the enormous tension between India and Pakistan, Daddy's family finally decided to emigrate to the UK in hope of a better, more stable future. They departed on a large passenger ship that was headed for Southampton, UK. It was 20 October 1956 when Daddy, who was eleven years old, embarked on their seventeen-day journey with his family from Asia to Europe. He told us how they boarded the ship from Karachi, passing by Yemen, the Suez Canal, the Mediterranean, Malta, Gibraltar, and the Bay of Biscay.

Daddy told us how the passenger ship was a luxury liner

carrying about 2000 people. He particularly enjoyed eating cornflakes cereal from the breakfast buffet. This obviously meant something to Daddy because the cereal cupboard at home never failed to have cornflakes in it. He said people received table numbers telling them where to sit at mealtimes. This continued to be important to him because our family usually sat and ate together whenever we were at home.

At the time when Daddy was passing through the Suez Canal with his family, there was a conflict going on between some countries. By 5 November, Britain and France had landed paratroopers along the Suez Canal. Before the Egyptian forces were defeated, they managed to sink forty ships in the canal, which resulted in the canal being blocked. Daddy explained how, by chance, the ship he was on with his family was one of the last ships that passed through the Suez Canal before the bombardment began. The passengers didn't know that this was going on since they were not kept informed. It was only once the ship had been cleared from the Suez Canal that the passengers were told there was a conflict and blockade of the channel that the ship had narrowly avoided.

Daddy knew the ship had docked at Southampton Port during the night of 5 November and the early hours of 6 November, because it had been Guy Fawkes' Night[8] in Britain. He could see smoke across the sky from bonfires that had been burning the night before.

During this tense time, Dadajaan was still working in London at Saville Row as a tailor and cutter. He had been waiting anxiously in the UK for his family to arrive, while being naturally concerned, not knowing what was happening to them on their journey. Fortunately, they arrived on 6 November 1956, settling safely in London. Six years later, after arriving in the UK at the age of sixteen, Daddy had become a British citizen. I only have one vague memory of Dadajaan. It is from when I was around three years old and he had been sitting with us children as we ate some marmalade and cheese on toast together. It was rather tasty.

When Mum met Daddy

Mum's family decided to immigrate to Kuwait: a small but beautiful Arab country. Her Daddy had a hobby of riding horses there. When he had time, he travelled via the UK to visit my Dadajaan who made jockey clothing especially for him. Friendships are a wonderful thing, are they not? How great it was that no borders or boundaries stopped them from the chance to meet up!

I often asked Daddy how he met Mum because of my curiosity about how they got together. I wanted to know if he had been set up to marry her or not, especially because our culture was one where there were lots of arranged marriages. I didn't get the feeling that it would matter to me if it had been an arranged marriage since, from what I could see from my uncles and Aunties around me, they seemed to get on fine. It turns out the relationship was described as a "love marriage." This phrase stuck in my mind whenever I saw Mum and Daddy being romantic with each other. We listened avidly each time he told us the same story about how they met.

It was March 1971 when Mum's grandfather took his family to visit some of his children who were living in Canada. Mum who was around twenty-years-old at the time, joined the family for this journey, which was from Kuwait to Canada via transit in the UK. Transiting via London meant that Mum's grandfather got a chance to visit Dadajaan because they knew each other from Pakistan. Mum didn't stay at Daddy's home, but the families had plenty to talk about, easily finding reasons to meet up. This was the first chance Daddy got to spend time with Mum because he had been asked to take her shopping. Daddy said he was excited to spend this time with Mum even though it was only for a week.

Daddy carried on telling us the story, saying, "When you set your eye on someone for the first time, it's an instant feeling". Then, he smiled saying, "It went the way I wanted," since he found out that she liked him back. Daddy said that the interest was mutual, but of course back then, approval had to follow from each family.

Mum went on to Canada, heading back to Kuwait earlier than the rest of her family because of her college studies. During her travel back to Kuwait from Canada, she was allowed to transit via London again.

All South Asians know that they are requested, if not expected, to collect family from the Airport by car upon arrival in the country. Since Daddy worked at London Heathrow Airport, he gladly collected Mum while dutifully driving her to his auntie's home where she stayed for a few days. At the end of her stay, he put her safely on her flight back home to Kuwait. The interest between the two was mutual, resulting in engagement after swift approval between Mum's grandfather and Dadajaan.

Daddy visited Mum's family in Kuwait to meet them all. Mum had prepared a traditional sweet dish for him called Samia (which is vermicelli), but because it was made in Kuwait, where a mixed array of seeds are used in dishes, it had cardamom mixed with sliced almonds in it. He told me that he liked the taste of it very much, hitting exactly the right spot, which means it went straight to his heart. I knew that warm feeling in the heart from when I got some good home-cooked food that had been passed onto me and was not surprised that it was there at the beginning of Mum and Daddy's love story.

Mum cooked a few variations of Pakistani dishes when she had visits from the Asian community. Whether it was friends from Yemen, Pakistan, or India, they all commented on how they liked the difference in taste. This must have been the influence she got from learning to cook in Kuwait. Everybody loved Mum's cooking. It only took six months from Mum and Daddy meeting each other in March to the engagement in May until the wedding in August. After the wedding, Mum and Daddy travelled back to the UK to live their lives together.

Upon arrival in the UK at London Heathrow Airport, they showed the marriage certificate from Kuwait to the immigration officers. Daddy was asked if he was employed, to which he replied yes. He confirmed that he was working as a ground support services engineer for the airline industry at BOAC, the British Overseas Airways Corporation that eventually became British Airways. His job at London Heathrow Airport meant he had to take care of all the machinery that was used to support the aircraft. Daddy's employment in the UK was all that he was asked to confirm when he came back to the UK with Mum. Mum, on the other hand, wasn't asked anything.

Daddy lived on Killarney Road with his parents and his entire family together with Mum until my oldest brother, Abbid, was two years old. Then he found a house for his little family of three to settle into. I can imagine that living independently from his family, including his seven siblings, must have been quite exciting for him and Mum.

Chapter 3
Life with the A & A's

Changing Careers

Daddy became a mechanical engineer after his apprenticeship at British Airways at London Heathrow Airport. He worked on the ground fleet, checking the safety of vehicles, for quite a few years. In 1984, he decided to do something different, so he ran a petrol station for about a year.

After a short time working there, he decided with Mum to open a retail business in the form of - yes, you guessed it - (like many South Asians who emigrated over to the UK) a corner shop. It was called A&A's Mini-Mart. The name represented the family, since each of our names started with the letter A.

Working together to run a family business was a big change. With it came opportunities, but also challenges. Now Daddy was self-employed, which gave him the freedom to be his own boss. This also put him under pressure to bring in his own income. The advantage was that my parents could spend more time together than when Daddy had been working at the Airport. A typical day at the shop involved Daddy waking up at 5:30 am, driving to the shop, and loading up the car full of items that local small businesses had pre-ordered. He would usually have all of this done by 7:30 am, in time to prepare to open the shop for his customers.

Customers came in each morning, buying the morning newspaper to read on their way to work. The shop had a steady flow of students and staff coming in at lunchtime from the local college opposite the shop. This continued until the college management decided to create a huge gate. The gate was constantly closed, making it hard for students or staff to pass through to where the shop was, thereby killing off a big part of the shop's income. Of course this impacted him as a family man trying to feed a family of four kids.

Sometimes, after dropping us off at school, Mum would come to the shop at around 10:00 am with breakfast for Daddy, telling him to go to the stock room at the back to eat it in peace while she took care of running the shop. Daddy used this time to get stock during the day. Daddy would then come back to the shop, leaving Mum to pick us up from school. This husband-and-wife teamwork meant that the family could all be together at home by 7:30 pm instead of 9:30 pm.

Sometimes, I watched how customers handled the fruit. Before finally deciding not to buy it, they would come in, pick it up, squeeze it, and throw it up into the air until it landed in their hands, before putting it back again. He would tell the customers not to touch it unless they were going to buy it. I watched with Mum to see how they reacted. Of course, once the fruit was bruised, no one wanted to buy it, which meant Daddy brought it home so it wasn't wasted. Although I complained at the time that we never got the fresh, good stuff, the idea that Daddy didn't want the food to go to waste stayed with me.

Daddy would usually ring us at the end of each day to check if there were essentials we needed. We often slipped in the request for chocolate - not sugar-boiled sweets, but chocolate. We definitely had our fair share, but my teeth are still pretty good.

Tricky Times

Around that time, Daddy would get phone calls at home from the police saying that the shop alarm had gone off due to a burglary. Even though Daddy removed the cigarettes and alcohol from the front of the shop into a secure stock room, those items were predominantly what people seemed to want to steal. One of the strangest ways someone had thought up to break in, was by driving a small Mini Cooper car into the front of the shop.

Each time a break-in happened, which was quite a few times, unfortunately, it was upsetting. So much time, effort, and cost were involved in managing those situations. Mum would sit with us while we waited to hear from Daddy about what had happened when he came home. I remember the upset look on his face. It made me think twice about being self-employed because of the distress it caused.

Mum and Daddy always knew how much to charge for items according to a book that had all the prices in it. There was also a small book for IOUs that was used to keep track of customers who were unable to pay immediately. They would note down the IOU of what was owed, then cross it off once it got paid by the customer, who would come in saying, "I Owe You" to pay what was owed. Daddy had a trust-based agreement, which over time showed me that sometimes you win, but sometimes you lose.

I used to work at the shop occasionally with Aneesa, helping to break down boxes for the rubbish collection, compacting the empty boxes that had already been unpacked. I took one box to crush and rammed my foot against it hard, thinking it was empty. Then, I heard a crunch. I realised that it wasn't empty at all. I laughed my head off with Aneesa, but Daddy wasn't impressed. I felt bad after realising I had almost destroyed a completely unopened box of mints. Our playful antics as twins didn't stop when we were teenagers. In fact, there was always something we could laugh about in between work and studying.

We would chat with customers from the old people's home up the road who would come to the shop just to get outside. Sometimes we would walk them back to their homes so they had company. Occasionally they would come in to buy something from the shop when they were only interested in a chat. It would make me laugh when they found something funny. Once or twice, laughing made their false teeth fall out.

"Hello there, Jazz," they would say to Daddy. "Ooh, your daughters are here." Then they would chat with us girls for a while since they had plenty of time on their hands.

"He's lovely; your Dad is. He helps me get in and out of the shop, he does. He walks me across the road to the corner." Then they would chuckle with laughter running out of breath, like people who let themselves spurt out laughter after a good giggle do. We would stand there with our eyes wide open, trying not to laugh until we headed back to the stock room, giggling from seeing their false teeth fall out. I realised later it was better to laugh together with someone rather than at them.

Mixed Cultures

Daddy had created a great sense of community by running his corner shop. It felt like the shop was a hub where locals would come in to get the essential items they needed. It became a place where laughter mixed with tears were shared by customers. Sometimes Black customers from the West Indies would come in. They would give us a nod, raising their hand to say hello by saying "Alright" stretching the letter "I" when they said the word. It sounded like they were saying "Alriiiiiiight." Their accents were something I really loved hearing. They would often go for the super malt drink at the back of the shop.

The Asian customers would order samosas, telling my Dad to compliment the cook about how tasty they were. They would ask, "Are they fresh, uncle? Are they fresh?" The English customers would grab a cheese and onion or steak and kidney Cornish pasty. There was something for most of the communities that passed through to put a smile on their faces. Most importantly for me, I got to try different foods from different cultures. The mixed wave of cultures of people passing through the shop made me see how people can co-exist while going about their daily lives peacefully.

Once, a couple of young boys came in, seriously arguing with each other. Daddy had known them since they were little kids, but now they were young boys. One pulled out a knife to threaten the other. Daddy wasn't having any of that in his shop. He got in between them to stop the fight, getting his hand cut in the process. The mother of one of the boys came by later to thank him for stepping in to break up the fight. Those stories scared me because we would worry about his safety at the shop.

Daddy's safety would be at risk simply by him trying to intervene and prevent someone getting hurt in the shop. I was afraid he would not come home at all one day. It made me think twice about whether or not to intervene if I should ever see a fight break out, because people are irrational or violent when they are angry. Would I be the bystander, or would I also step in like Daddy did? Working at the shop meant dealing with the public. It meant every day there was the risk of something happening that was unpredictable. Working in an office provides you with a completely different sort of safety and risk.

We would talk to the customers a little, but generally, I would find myself reading the magazines or newspapers while avoiding eye contact with the top shelf, which was lined with magazines for the over eighteens. Mum happily read the UK newspapers along with the Urdu or Arabic ones, which meant she was fully up to date with what was going on in different parts of the world that she once grew up in.

Sometimes, kids would come in with a list from their parents, who had given them money to buy their groceries. If they tried to buy cigarettes or alcohol, Daddy would point them straight to the notice saying, "Over 18's Only." He told them what the consequences could be for him if he sold items to underage customers. He explained how he could lose his license to sell alcohol in his shop. They would walk away looking sheepish or irritated or defeated from not having gotten what they wanted. The fact that Daddy had to explain it to them showed me that either their parents didn't know what their children got up to, or the parents just didn't care. This made me realise that, even though parents could be really strict sometimes, it was because they had a responsibility to teach their children the difference between right and wrong.

Most of the customers were harmless, but sometimes they were drunk, if not a little aggressive. I would watch Mum calmly let them say what they wanted in the hope that they wouldn't stay too long. When those customers came into the shop, Mum would tell us in Punjabi to go to the stockroom immediately, which we did. I kept an eye out through the door to check if she was safe. Once the bothersome customer had gone, one of us would open the shop door to get some fresh air inside, to remove the tension in the air that was still lingering.

I wasn't worried that anything would happen to Mum, but in those situations, I had the urge to check she was ok. Mum was absolutely fine and I never ever saw her have to raise her voice or become aggressive. I guess those characteristics followed me because I saw later on in life that it would take a lot for me to get angry or explode. Sometimes there are other ways to let out your frustration. I think Mum would have been proud with how we handled ourselves in difficult situations. I was just sorry she wasn't there to telephone so that I could listen to her voice when I had something to tell her.

We had dishonest customers too. Sometimes they would pay, hand over money, and then say how they had given a twenty-pound note when they had only given ten. I watched my parents learn from those situations by perching myself on the side stool while they served tricky customers. Daddy would take the customer's money, saying out loud, "That's £10," or "That's £20." He kept the bank note in his hand in full view of the customer or left the money on top of the cash register, until the difference owed to the customer had been given back to them. Then he placed the cash into the cash register. The looks on their faces when they realised they couldn't get away with their behaviour made me form an early opinion about honesty in people versus those who want to see what they could get away with.

One customer who used to come in drunk for many years spent a long time talking to Daddy. Many years later, when she saw us twins in the shop, she told us how our Daddy had convinced her to not buy the cider in a big bottle, but instead, he gave her a huge bag of oranges. She told us how he helped save her which led to her becoming sober. That made me feel proud of my Daddy because it showed me that he cared about his customers.

Whether it was Daddy telling children that they couldn't buy items for Over 18's only, or breaking up a fight with teenagers, or being a good Samaritan and helping someone to become sober, it showed me a perspective of how to behave in life. I appreciated the importance of sticking together as a family, and being on guard in case someone was in trouble.

Pilgrimage to Mecca and Medina

In the 1980s, Daddy worked abroad as a contractor for a few months at a time, at Jeddah Airport in Riyadh, the capital of Saudi Arabia. He earned more money, which certainly helped with raising four children. During that time, while Mum ran the shop, Daddy's mum helped by taking us to school. I don't remember the goodbyes when Daddy went to work abroad, but when he came back, I knew it was him because of the way he rang the doorbell. We would run downstairs full of excitement, seeing him standing there with his suitcase.

We didn't go on holiday very often. Instead we spent our time visiting relatives at the weekend, which was usually fun. In fact, we only went abroad a couple of times, ever. Once was to Disney World in Florida. The other time was to Saudi Arabia.

We arrived at Mecca, the holy place for Muslims. It was daylight. The entrance was lined with many poor or needy people who sat begging. It was probably the first time I ever saw people who were less able or fortunate than me asking for money. Mum explained to me how they were allowed to accept money from those more fortunate than they were. That meant we were fortunate, so we gave some money to them. It showed me what being charitable meant. I realised then that many people had been dealt a different set of cards in their life.

I gained completely new impressions from this foreign country that was so very different to my home in England. I grew up in the UK in a British-Asian household, but this was an Arab country that was completely unfamiliar to me. Seeing the Arab people dressed in their traditional clothes was an eye-opener.

I felt like I had to behave the whole time because there were so many guards in uniform who all looked very serious. Their presence at guarding the area made me feel like I was somewhere important. It was a bit like when you see the guards at Buckingham Palace in London protecting the building. If you upset them or got too close, they stamped their feet hard on the ground and shouted out loud telling you to stand back. That wasn't the time to be silly and play around. I never felt scared or unsafe because of the guards since Mum was always there protecting me. Today I feel protected by Mum but in a different way. I feel like she is around me, albeit not in the physical form.

The space was so huge that I could see the Kaaba, the giant

black cube, from quite far away. We followed Mum as she started to walk around it. Mum kept us close, because so many people were walking around it all at the same time. One of the corners of the Kaaba had a huge stone on it that people tried to reach up to touch. It was quite high up above me. When I was near it, by chance a guard helped me touch the stone. Although the meaning remained vague to me, I remember feeling like the cool kid doing it.

Everyone moved in one direction around the big cube. There was special holy water we tasted called Zamzam water. This water had a softer texture to it. The smell in the air was different from what I was used to at home in the UK. It consisted of a mixture of dry air and a cool breeze, but without that cold, bitter feeling I knew from the UK where the chill got to my bones. It was quite different from what I knew.

We went on a drive from Mecca to Medina which is a journey people do on this sort of trip. Medina has a mosque where the Prophet Muhammad is buried. You could regularly hear out loud the call to prayer, which was heard throughout the day. We were inside Medina Sharif Mosque in the area that was for women only. It was one of the many occasions where it was only us girls with Mum. The space wasn't particularly stylish inside the mosque; in fact, it was very plain. The only material thing to touch was the carpet on the ground, which had a soft feel to it. The impression I got at the time was that nothing gold or glamourous needed to be displayed in a place of prayer where the only importance was your connection with God.

It was daytime when we visited, but being inside meant it wouldn't have mattered what time of day or night it was. Inside, the lighting was calm, without too much emphasis on colour or ornaments, as I would have expected. I felt comfortable because Mum was taking care of her girls. She made sure we were kept close by her side. I felt the motherly love when she took our hands tightly, holding them whenever we walked around unknown places, or when we sat next to her, which happened often. I felt safe and comfortable amidst the hive of strangers rushing about, speaking unfamiliar languages. It gave me a feeling of stability knowing she was there as our protector.

She sat relaxed, with her body poised in such a way that she was taking her attendance there seriously. Because Mum grew up in Kuwait, her Arabic was fluent. For us girls, we didn't understand any of it, although we had learned the first few letters of the Arabic alphabet: Alif, Baa, Taa, Tha. Mum read the Quran out loud but quietly while we sat listening. Her voice had a high-pitched soft gentle sound, never attracting attention. Simply hearing her voice gave me a calm feeling, which made me feel grounded. That sound sits with me in my heart. I can still hear her voice when I think about her.

I remembered how when we did prayers at home in Reading, us kids would sometimes start giggling because we couldn't sit still. Mum would start the prayer, stopping to tell us off because we were being disrespectful. In these moments, we had to start all over again, trying not to laugh. We tried to focus but got a bout of giggles again, resulting in us having to start over once more. I have said it before, and I'll say it again, we were very cheeky twins. Now I was somewhere foreign, behaving impeccably to avoid getting lost amongst the masses of people. The mere idea of being separated from Mum terrified me. She was extra vigilant about our whereabouts, and although she could spot us in a crowd, her outfit was black like almost every other woman around us.

The sound of the holy prayer in Medina could be heard all over the city through speakers. It was interesting, not like a singing sound, but a rhythmic melody that always had a man's voice. I wondered what it might be like to hear a woman announce the call to prayer. It's a sound I had never heard. My imagination took me to a calm place where the sound of the women's voices bellowed across the vast valleys of a made-up place in my head. I suspect that if I were to hear it someday, I would like it. I am quite sure it would make me reflect, feeling happy that women are leading the prayer and being visible.

At some point, a group of women came to sit right in front of us. One of them could see Mum reciting the Quran quietly and could hear her. She approached Mum, asking if she could read the Quran to them since no one in their group could read Arabic. Mum gladly did it for them. That was the first time I experienced what it felt like to be proud. I was proud of my cool Mum.

The women were all dressed in black from top to toe. So was Mum. This was the first time I saw her fully dressed in traditional Arab clothing. She had never dressed like this at home in the UK. We didn't dress in black since we were only young girls at the time, so there was no expectation for us to do so. The women's faces were visible, but the rest of them was covered. Although, outside, that was how almost all the women looked, I had never actually sat amongst a group of women all dressed the same before. It felt completely foreign being around them, but it was nice seeing how happy they were, and all because they were being helped by my Mum. Yes, my modest Mum, who was happy to help those strangers. Not showing off or speaking too loudly; she formed a connection with them for that short time. I had a feeling this small encounter left a lasting impression on them. Mum seemed to connect well with other women regardless of whether it was in Saudi or at home in her Asian community, and as I got older, I realised how having a sense of community mattered to me too.

I realised then, being amongst these women, what a sense of community felt like. I didn't form any judgements back then about how everyone was dressed. I guessed they were used to it whereas I wasn't. It was foreign to me, which made sense because I was somewhere different to what I was used to. My impression of them was that they were strong, confident women. They were respectful toward each other. Most importantly, for me, I didn't feel uncomfortable. Mum was totally relaxed about it. She was happy she could help them. It's probably the first time I'd seen what it feels like to help others who you don't know. I was gushing in admiration for my Mum who was the person doing the helping.

I saw how saying goodbye wasn't simply in the form of a handshake. It was a lean into the cheek on the left, then the right. Then it was another lean into the left again, finishing with the right again. We quietly giggled, watching on. When would we ever get home, I wondered, after seeing how long it took to say goodbye this way to everyone. I learned over the years that it takes about half an hour to say goodbye when you are ready to depart your attendance somewhere that involves Asians or Arabs. It's certainly warmer than a polite handshake, but two steps away from a warm hug.

That evening, while we were waiting in the car for Daddy to bring back some samosas for us to eat before the journey back to Jeddah, Mum started to introduce us to our first-ever prayers in Arabic. When she spoke them out loud to us, we repeated the words back to her. She took time to correct us with the pronunciation of how the words sounded. Eventually, the words rippled off my tongue easily. After memorising the prayers, I visualised myself doing a small success dance. I took a sip of 7 Up from a small glass bottle. I will never forget how good it tasted. I don't know if the ingredients were different, or if it tasted so good because it was refreshing in comparison to the warm dry air outside. All I know is that back home in Reading, I couldn't conjure up that refreshing taste again, the one I remembered from that time when we were in Saudi Arabia with Mum and Daddy.

Arabian Adventures

Saudi Arabia was one of the countries my parents got married in, so they were familiar with it. Plus, being in an Arab country probably meant Mum was in her comfort zone with the culture. While Daddy was working, Mum cooked for the family. We played outside in a courtyard which wasn't your average English-style courtyard with a wooden fence or a red brick wall. There was stone that was in its natural form from our feet leading all the way up above us to a rock edge. We could see goats at the top pushing stones over the edge that fell from the top down to where we were playing. At night, there was the constant sound of crickets chirping. I still have the sound of them in my mind today. They could be heard singing all night.

Daddy drove us around in his Honda Accord, which had velvet curtains at the back to stop the heat from outside coming through. He had the Honda transported to the UK and it happened to be the first car I learned to drive in.

My first memory of going to a beach was in Saudi Arabia. It was exciting. I was completely fascinated by the sea life, the corals, or the starfish since I had never seen them in the UK. I was absorbed by the different things I found on the beach, not noticing how the water had started to run over my small feet. I held a starfish in my young hand. It felt rough to touch. The piece of coral I found was even larger. It was a very strong white colour. Its texture wasn't smooth but touching something different for the first time felt exciting.

I heard Mum calling me from afar, telling me to hurry back. I looked up, smelling sea air, following the sound of Mum's voice calling my name. I could only make out her blurry shadow because of the bright sunlight. I carried on looking deeper into what had caught my eye. I probably wasn't that far out from the shore, but I was far out enough for her to be worried.

Mum called out for me again to come back quickly, which I immediately did. I dropped the coral, quickly put down the starfish that I had spent ages staring at, fascinated by its colourful shape, all the while making sure I didn't damage it. When I got to Mum, she grabbed my hand tightly, pulling me towards her. She walked quickly with me back to the dry part of the beach. She didn't tell me off, but she wasn't happy that I had wandered off so far. I learned to watch out for Mum's stern look in her eyes and understood it as a silent expression of disappointment. That feeling made my eyes expand and my heart sink in an instant over the years when I upset her.

Leaving the sea water when it was rising up after Mum called me, somehow gave me a cautious feeling of going into water. Mum must have noticed this. I think she wanted her children to overcome our hesitation of being in water. When we got back from Saudi Arabia, she arranged for us to have swimming lessons before having them at school. She watched us from the side, not being able to swim herself, but always encouraged us. That made me feel close to her and safe.

I never questioned that we would be together for many decades more, naively assuming there would be hundreds of more occasions to show her what we had learned, be it in water, skiing, or rock climbing. I still send videos to Daddy, but I know he would have loved to share them with Mum.

Chapter 4
A Glorious Childhood

The Twin Effect

Once we moved from Maidenhead to Reading, Berkshire, us twins continued to have violin lessons. The only violin teacher available was at another school nearby so we had to have our lessons there. One day we had accidentally 'forgotten' our violins at home which, I am pretty certain, was because we didn't like going to the school nearby for lessons. When the Headmistress found out we had forgotten them, she walked us home to get them. I don't know why she did it, but it made me feel special. I realised then that we were liked by the teachers who looked out for us identical twins. It's probably because we put a smile on their faces from being happy, sensible girls who listened to our teachers, rather than cheeky rascals who irritated them. They saw the effort Mum made with our school uniforms by adding flowery bow ties for us to wear. The headmistress complimented us twins on how impressive we looked, and we would relay that back to Mum who loved hearing what we told her. Then she would change our hair clips and bring a bit more colour into our hair styles. Perhaps it was because we had bundles of energy. We easily spoke to each other twice as fast as we did to anyone else.

Hair, So Much Hair

Mum loved making sure we were dressed presentably because people often stared at us twins. She spent a fair bit of time combing our long hair. We would sit for ages while she combed it, trying out different styles on us both, never tiring from it. We just wanted to move around, which is what little girls want to do, rather than sit still for an eternity. We sat there for what felt like hours on end as she adjusted it, using different coloured ribbons, clips, or feathers. The strength in her fingers was notable while she braided our hair. Her fingers knew exactly how our hair was formed, what direction it went in, or what pressure to apply to get a style to stay in place. Mum loved having her twin girls to do girly things with. I think she loved having girls because she could relate to being female herself. She spent a considerable amount of time putting make up on us until we could do it ourselves. Every now and then all three of us dressed the same, which felt really special.

When we were eight years old, our school took us to have swimming lessons at the local pool. Preparing our very long hair to fit into the swimming cap was particularly difficult. Mum would separate our long, dark black hair that went down to our bottoms into four parts with a comb, somehow squeezing it all compactly into the rubber swimming cap. After the lesson we would get home to wash the chlorine from the water out of our hair. We would take out the ribbons from our braids; by now frizzy and full of tangles. I hated that part, but had to do it in order to learn to swim.

For one of our birthdays, an uncle of mine wanted to gift us a haircut, thinking we could do with a style that wasn't long hair. He gave us a magazine with a range of different hair styles to choose from. Mum was not impressed at all. We didn't get our long thick hair cut by a hairdresser on that occasion, or on any occasion while we were living at home.

Sometimes when Daddy got home from work, we would plead with him to comb our hair instead of Mum. He rarely did that; never interfering with how Mum raised us children, but he did do it twice where he gently combed it with the brush for about two strokes before passing the comb back for Mum to continue. Daddy probably knew he wouldn't do as good a job as Mum. Combing his twin girls' hair wasn't something he was familiar with, and he never went against Mum when it came to things at home that she usually took responsibility for. In a way, he showed us indirectly that he respected Mum by not taking over and undermining her.

Mum took pride in the things she did. I watched her plant roses in the garden which smelled lovely. She often pottered around in the garden wearing her gardening gloves to plant flowers or strawberries or more roses. I could see she loved her roses, taking her time to prune them. The roses travelled with us to whichever house we lived in, bringing colour and scented smells into each garden in which they were planted. The rose bushes were the one constant thing that didn't change even though almost everything else did. We all grew older, as did the roses, but while they stayed in the garden, we moved up to the new school, making new friends along the way. What we didn't expect was that life would soon change in such a dramatic way for us because of Mum.

The Life of Musicality and Sports

Aged eleven, we had started life at secondary school. We spent most of our time in the music and drama, or sports departments. I never failed to feel protected by Mum. When I was in my first year of secondary school, there was an away match, so we had to take the bus to get there. On the way back, I sat at the back thinking it was free for all seating. Actually, it's where most girls from the year above sat. They were having none of it, telling me in no unclear terms that it wasn't meant for my year group to sit there. I responded saying, "Oh, really? What are you going to do about it?"

At that moment, one of them grabbed me by the back of my shirt, digging her knuckles into my back so it hurt. I sat there, holding back my tears while my shirt was being grabbed. When I got into the car where Mum was waiting, I burst into tears, telling her what had happened. With that, she went to talk to the sports teacher, who then irritatingly came over to the car, immediately telling me off for not going to her directly.

The next morning, the school organised an assembly on the topic of how bullying would not be tolerated at school. I was quite surprised. The girl had to apologise to me, which she did. She said she only did it because the sports teacher who took us on the trip was the only teacher she liked. I was fine with her apology. What this showed me was how the school took bullying seriously, at least on this occasion. Mum, my protector, was ready to step in because I couldn't handle doing something about the incident myself. I wasn't embarrassed and learned later as an adult that if it's appropriate and necessary, you should do the same. You don't let someone suffer if they tried but need help.

From then on, you couldn't keep me off the sports grounds. Whether it was hockey, netball, tennis, the discus, or shot put, I was there. I lived and breathed the sports and music departments while I was at school. I would spend hours playing team sports, composing music, playing in an orchestra, or singing in a choir. That was the fun-filled life I had. Sports helped me work in teams, while music was a great way to be creative. Plus, all the cool kids were either doing sports or music or drama.

While eating disorders like anorexia began to take hold of some of my school mates, I failed to notice whether I stayed the same size. I didn't think much about how I looked in my school uniform. Being happy was more important. Mum wanted us to be well-presented, but she never commented on our size. It didn't seem important to her. A standard week before and after school for us twins comprised of the following:

MONDAY 8 AM TO 9 AM: AMNESTY CHOIR.
This Amnesty choir was brilliant to sing in. At a school

assembly, we watched a couple of students sing Imagine by John Lennon. I was so impressed with the sound, but also with the performance being in front of the whole school. My connection with music changed after that. I ended up in the Amnesty choir, where I was lucky enough to sing with some of the older kids. We sang *No Milk Today* by Graham Gouldman. I heard what boys sounded like when they sang alto, tenor or even bass. It was enriching to my ears.

There were no prejudices based on age in that choir. In fact, there were no prejudices at all. It was all focused on the sound of music. Mum was proud that her twin girls were singing in yet another choir. We would get home after school to find ourselves singing away in the kitchen regularly while Mum was making dinner. I think she liked listening to her twins sing. Perhaps it was because when she grew up in Kuwait, she learned to dance in a style called Kathak which looked difficult to do. I had seen photos of how happy she looked as she was learning the dance. I know studying and doing well was extremely important to Mum and Daddy, and most Asian parents, but how lucky we were that our parents let us express ourselves through all the music we did.

MONDAY AFTER SCHOOL: VIOLIN LESSONS.

How we came to play the violin was a bit odd. We were sitting in a school assembly. I wasn't listening to what was being said by the headmaster. For some reason, my older brother stood up. Without knowing why he did that, the headmaster then asked everyone, "Anyone else?" So we both stood up too because we saw him do it. We knew from Mum to listen to our brother because he was the eldest, and in that moment something inside told me to listen to him and do what he was doing, so I did, as did Aneesa. As it turned out, we had just signed up to take music lessons like our older brother. We were then taken to a room that was full of orchestral instruments, including violins. I went over picking one for myself. It was a half-size violin, although I eventually got a full-size one after growing a bit taller.

Playing the violin was a gift, as was music in itself. It led to us playing Pachelbel's Canon in D with the orchestra. I played *"The Arrival of the Queen of Sheba"* by George Friederic Handel, and Mozart's *"Eine Kleine Nachtmusik"*. I got to play this wonderful music all thanks to a wonderful mistake of following my instinct of not leaving Abbid to stand up on his own. Those harmonies were beautiful; the melodies rich when heard in an orchestra. Those classical pieces remain imprinted in my mind, making me feel nourished.

TUESDAY 8 AM: SINGING LESSONS.
There was a yearly carnival in the area we lived in where one of the choirs I sang in was performing. I sang a duet with Aneesa at the carnival, when out of the blue, a lady asked us if we would be interested in singing at an old people's home because she was impressed with what she had heard. Being twins must have helped too. People seemed to be excited by our voices sounding identical. We got paid £200 for singing. That wasn't bad for a first paid performance, was it?

The funniest part was when we finished singing "Yesterday" by the Beatles. After asking the residents if they had any requests, they immediately said they wanted to hear "Yesterday" by the Beatles. Memory is such a fascinating thing. To retain it is a gift. To lose it is a tragedy. Was Mum proud of us for being asked to sing to others outside of school? Yes, she was.

WEDNESDAY 8 AM: ORCHESTRA FOLLOWED BY RECORDER ENSEMBLE AFTER SCHOOL.
We went to Mockbeggar House, an old house that was available for teaching music. The house looked huge from the outside, but the sounds that were produced in it were incredible to hear. It's where I sat my grade 5 music theory exam with

Aneesa. It's where we played the recorders, learned about the treble and bass clef. It's where we realised that if we didn't start practicing our musical instruments soon, we would not be able to advance in our lives as musicians. That's why we sat down, studied music theory, and took the Associated Board of Music exams, passing with an identical result of 85% each. Our music theory teachers were quite shocked at our results. Of course we were too, leaving us bursting with pride at our achievement.

Who would have thought us cheeky kids could take something so seriously while performing so well? It showed the others how it was possible to succeed when you studied hard enough. Without encouragement from our teachers, we wouldn't have made it. One must hold onto the encouragement that a teacher gives, because when one hits the working world, it doesn't come in droves.

THURSDAY EVENINGS: JUDO.

Who would have imagined that our Asian parents would have been cool about us girls learning self-defence at such a young age? I started Judo with Aneesa before my younger brother who began a little later than us. This sport, being one of defence, not attack, taught me about discipline, team participation, and competition. Mum would watch us come home from judo lessons all excited about having learned how to defend ourselves.

When she took us to competitions at the local sports centre, she would watch us compete, standing by, ready to cheer us on. "Come on, Aisha, come on, Aneesa," she would say when we had to fight against each other. She was clearly our biggest fan. She was proud when we came home with a medal or even a trophy.

We became pretty good at Judo, which led us to competing internationally in Germany twice. It was an exciting time for us kids since we grew up in a strict, disciplined household. Being allowed to travel outside of the family set-up was a huge deal in those days. Our judo teachers had several conversations with my parents and even came to our house to reassure them that we would be supervised, which we were. I don't know how Mum was fine with us going to Germany at the age of 14, but when something involved adult supervision, she was open-minded enough to let her girls participate. It's something Aneesa and I were always grateful for.

There were a few funny moments where Mum had telephoned to check that we had arrived safely. We sat chatting away in the evening with our hosts, who were also twins - yes, we had been paired with twins – when suddenly their mother came in with the phone, wearing not much more than a small top over her lingerie. We nearly burst into hysterics because we had grown up in an Asian household where, even though I shared a room with my twin, we turned around when we were changing clothes. It just was like that. Yet here was a stranger totally comfortable with however she was dressed in her own home. We stared at her with our big brown eyes wide open, trying not to look shocked. I told Mum afterwards about what we saw. She was quite surprised too, but she could see the funny side.

It was an eye opener into a different culture, showing me rules and boundaries are different based on where one is living in the world. These people were more relaxed at home when it came to their bodies and clothing. Even though I felt British Asian growing up, I had grown up in a home with the boundaries of an Asian girl, and even though they say, "When in Rome do as the Romans do", I was not going to be seen doing the same either in Germany, or at home, and I was absolutely fine with that. There were enough other women I could think of who would never have let their girls spend time outside of the family home, let alone abroad in a non-Asian or non-British culture. I felt extremely lucky and privileged that our parents agreed to us having this experience. Hoorah to my Mum and Daddy who let us go.

My Mum was strict but open-minded. She raised us to literally defend ourselves against others. I explained to school friends what moves we had learned in Judo to defend ourselves, such as an armlock, a choke or a strangle but I never actually tried anything out on them because that was against the rules. You don't do Judo outside of the Judo mat unless you have to use it in defence. Mum listened in but didn't comment. She had seen how we worked things out on our own ever since we climbed the bathroom cabinet as toddlers. I had the feeling she was preparing us girls to be able to protect ourselves, to know the difference between what was right and wrong in daily life, because we all know, sometimes parents can't be there to protect you, can they? Aneesa had quite a bad injury during a judo match where someone had thrown her in the air while putting her into an arm lock on her elbow at the same time. It was practically impossible for her to tap to surrender, thereby stopping the match. When she told Mum what had happened, Mum quickly stepped into action as Supermum. Whilst listening to Aneesa carefully describe where the pain was, she proceeded to quickly heat up some turmeric – an Asian spice – into a paste. She applied it carefully to Aneesa's elbow, wrapping it up firmly in cling film for it to heal. Then, the magic happened.

"There you go, *Beti* (daughter in Urdu), keep that on there," was her instruction. Over time, the turmeric, which reduced the inflammation in the arm, reduced the pain. I mean, making homemade wax to get rid of body hair was one thing but using spices as medicine was a whole new level of having a mum full of smart ideas, especially when it worked. I was really impressed with how Mum helped Aneesa's injury heal. She was back on the Judo mat fairly soon after that.

FRIDAY AFTER SCHOOL: ORCHESTRA.

I absolutely loved Friday night orchestra. It was such a highlight for us because it was at the end of the school week. The music sessions were held on our school grounds, again, providing my parents with reassurance of our safety. We had an orchestra conductor who reminded me of the Queen. She spoke rather eloquently and would conduct us with vigour while displaying her elegance at the same time. This fun for my soul mixed with the sounds we produced in the orchestra was just magnificent, in my opinion. I came away feeling enriched from the music, energised by the sounds, happy for the company and grateful we were allowed to go.

When we got picked up afterwards, a quick visit to the takeaway for fish and chips was the perfect way to end the week. Oh, how I loved that part of our evening: enjoying dinner with my family of six.

SATURDAY MORNINGS UNTIL 1PM: CHOIR.

On Saturday mornings we were at the Central Berkshire Music Centre where we had violin lessons, followed by junior orchestra and junior choir. Eventually we progressed to Friday night orchestra and girls' choir on Saturday mornings after which we would be picked up by Mum who waited patiently to bring us home.

The joy we got from music was carried through by my older brother Abbid and Aneesa who both conducted children's and adult choirs in their later lives. Taking Daddy along to concerts was good but also sad since over time he got used to sitting in the audience without Mum by his side. I am sure she would have loved to have been there to watch any of her children perform in later life; to be there like she had been when we were young, but she missed out on it.

What I noticed early on when I was a young girl was that when we went to Judo, there were no other Asian girls there.

When we went to school or to the music centre orchestra, there were no other Asian girls there either. Nor were there any other Asian girls when I sang in the school choirs. I realised how lucky we were to get to attend these activities that could have been seen as not the sorts of activities that Asian girls do.

We could have been told to stay at home to cook in the kitchen, which sometimes we did, but the balance was good for us. I think our parents wanted us to have opportunities that would help us develop into good people. Whatever the reason, I am grateful for all of what we had, and it's clearly my parents I must thank for that. I didn't miss seeing other Asian girls around since we met them at the community events for Asians, or at home, but I found it interesting that we were the only ones in some spaces.

Mum encouraging us to sing or play in front of an audience clearly helped us develop our confidence. We often ended up doing it with so much joy, that sometimes we jumped into action so fast that the guest audience was surprised. Clearly, we had been waiting for moments like this to perform all our lives.

I can confidently say it was thanks to Mum that our lives as teenagers were so rich. She watched over several cooking pots at once, making sure the temperature was right, or the ingredients were the correct measured amount. She watched over us in our teenage lives too where we were like a mixture of different pots full of music and arts; sports, or family events.

I am sure she discussed every activity her children did with Daddy, but ultimately it was because of her decisions that we grew up wearing traditional clothes at events and then came home being allowed to express ourselves with music or judo. I know that she put a lot of trust into the teachers who educated us at school or at the music centre. They were professional and looked after the students.

I believe it's because of the discussions her and Daddy had

with the adults about us being supervised, that we were given the freedom to enjoy so much throughout our teenage years at home. I also think at the back of my mind that our parents let us do all of these things to keep us away from hanging out after school with kids that may have led to us smoking or drinking or taking drugs. I don't think they even know that we didn't try any of that because we were far too busy being involved in our activities. I know Mum loved to do her Kathak dancing, and even belly dancing, and know she played the accordion, so perhaps she wanted us to have the same opportunities that she had in Kuwait until the age of 20. Yes, she had those opportunities too, and now she made sure we had the same chances as her.

Mum and Daddy were strict, and I think as long as we studied hard, and were good people respecting others, they were open to us learning how to play and even perform at a theatre school where three of us were in a performance of the *King and I*. They loved watching us at concerts and we loved performing. Surprisingly, we had mentioned wanting to go to Music Academy once we finished school, and neither Mum nor Daddy stopped us from talking to our teacher about it. As it turns out, we changed our minds after realising you had to be brilliant to get into the Royal Academy of Music.

What I realised was that we didn't go to a private school and yet we had the privilege to go to the music centre and have music lessons. If she were here now, I would have asked her why she felt it was acceptable for us to go when no other kids we knew from the South Asian background went. I have no idea if anyone from her community of women judged her for letting us girls go, and think she was really courageous for doing what felt right for her children and family. I do know, however, that when I spoke to some Asian girls at community events, they would say they weren't allowed to do what they wanted just because they were girls. It was in those moments that I thought how unfair it was being an Asian girl – for them at least.

Mum had a good way of teaching us how to look out for others. I knew that when she wasn't running the shop with Daddy, she was the perfect, typical housewife for an Asian family. She loved to cook, but also drove us around everywhere. Sometimes she would stop the car when an old person was crossing the road, telling us immediately to help them, which we gladly did with big smiles.

When I looked at Mum, I saw a strong-minded woman showing her kids how to be strong-minded too. She clearly played the biggest part in paving our way towards being confident girls.

Eclectic Edible Delights

Life as a teenager was so exciting. After Mum collected us, we would go home where food had been prepared. The smell of onions being fried together with garlic and ginger gave me such a cosy feeling when I got home. Stepping through the front door hungry for food, I would get a waft of the smell of onions being fried, making my mouth instantly water. I couldn't wait to eat what Mum had made for us.

Most of the kids we knew got three meals a day, but not us. For us, lunch time at school was a mammoth preparation task. Why could I never fit the apple, sandwiches, chocolate bar, crisps, and banana in my lunch box for school lunches? I would often sit with my school friends, offering something from the collection. Mum made sure we were able to share our food. We did that at school by asking our friends if they wanted one of our snacks.

It was much easier to share assorted chocolates than a solid chocolate bar, so we had an endless stream of friends, which felt great. Having friends, not only from school but also from our after-school activities, meant we had no shortage of people to invite to our birthday parties.

I was lucky to have had a fun, snack-filled childhood, which was normal for us kids back then. When friends came knocking on our door, we would invite them to chat away. Mum would bring us an Asian omelette with plain yoghurt and naan bread, which was an absolute favourite. It usually composed of eggs, chopped tomatoes, coriander, ginger, garam masala and onions. Everyone was happy. Mum, because she loved feeding us; our friends, because they got to try something different; and us twins because our friends were happy. We had no concept of any other kind of family life, which felt perfect growing up. It was fun, filled with happiness and love.

When we got home from school, when Mum was usually preparing dinner in the kitchen, we would talk about how our day went, while listening to her as she gave us advice. Many stories were told in the kitchen. I asked her about whether to use aerosols or roll-ons for deodorant, because of the huge hole in the earth's ozone layer above Australia caused by CFC (Chloroflurocarbon)emissions. The kitchen was where Mum gave us mother-daughter advice about who not to hang out with, how to respect our elders, how we were not designed to be vegetarians, how if a stranger who was my worst enemy arrived at my door, I should none the less offer them a glass of water, or how helping people in need was very important. If we wanted to go to a party, Mum would say, "Ask your father." Daddy would then say, "Ask your Mum." When I was older and moved out, I remembered those pearls of wisdom that Mum had given to me.

We watched her cook while taking instructions from her so we could help prepare dinner. "Aisha, get me some frozen ginger and garlic from the freezer." I would find it, bringing it over to her while she cut up tomatoes and onions for mixing in her blender. The large batches of fresh smelling coriander and mint would be cut by hand. Garam masala is a combination of ground spices that is most likely found in every South Asian kitchen. Garam means "hot" while the masala means "mixed spices." That's the key point. Usually, after a trip to Southall[9], Mum would get us to help her separate out the peel from cardamom pods. We would then gather the cumin seeds, coriander seeds, black peppercorns, cloves, cassia bark, and mustard seeds for her to make her own garam masala.

Whenever she finished blending the spices, I would see what the combination of them smelled like. Ooh, the smell gave me a feeling of being nourished - even nurtured because it came from Mum. I was absolutely convinced Mum's dishes tasted better than anyone else's meals because of the home made garam masala. And up to now, I haven't managed to recreate quite the same taste using the same mixture of spices in my Asian food. Daddy, on the other hand, has managed to replicate the taste of Mum's Asian omelette.

I didn't really like spicy food, but I did like food with spices. Daddy, on the other hand, was happy when Mum made a special side dish for him that had an entire fresh chili in it. We observed how Mum prepared the special version of the dish for Daddy in the kitchen. I watched in admiration, thinking about how much effort went into preparing each dish which took a fair bit of time to do. She made sure the seeds were separated by using the end of a knife to beat on the chili. That separated the seeds from the chili itself. She never touched the seeds with her hands. Then, she would add a whole green chili to the dishes for Daddy, who didn't mind eating them. In fact, he rather enjoyed his green chilis.

Mum always had special recipes or ingredients so could always try out something different. She loved cooking and I think it made her happy that we loved eating her food. With some instructions, we would prepare the dough from flour to make chapattis or roti, which my brothers loved eating very much. There was a fine line between the dough being the right consistency and having too much water in it. This meant sometimes that Mum had to rescue it to make it how it was meant to be. "Aisha, put some more flour in the bowl. Don't add too much water. Oh, give it here to me," Mum would say. "Sorry, Mum, it has too much water," would be my response.

It felt extra special when Mum made parathas filled with potatoes or minced meat. It took time to make them since they were usually two chapattis with a filling. I would stand watching Mum make them in the kitchen. It would start with her taking out the 10 kg bag of flour that was prepared for making the dough. Then the big heavy pan which looked like a semi-circle upside down wok, was placed over the gas fire. First butter was spread over the top of the pan with a kitchen towel. Then the chapatis were placed on top of the hot pan ready for cooking. The smell of cooked onions combined with spices inside the paratha made my mouth salivate. I waited patiently for the freshest paratha to land on the plate to share with Aneesa. The hot filling inside the paratha, eaten with fresh plain yoghurt, created an explosion of flavours inside my mouth. It's that intense smell of mixed spice, combined with the taste, that instantly took me back to feeling at home, surrounded by home-cooked food from Mum's kitchen.

The mincemeat chapati was usually one that Mum added fresh green chilies to. I knew it was going to be spicy chili hot. I would probably be shedding a few tears if I dared to try one. But I wanted to try them because they had been made by Mum so I knew they would taste good, but boy they were hot. I would eat the chapati with yoghurt to cool my mouth down when it was still burning. If that didn't work, I would eat a teaspoon of sugar or drink milk, which helped take off the heat.

Food played a major part in our lives. We got so much joy and satisfaction from eating together, be it with friends or family or at a restaurant to celebrate something. I learned that with cooking a curry, one has to have patience when preparing and not rush. Sometimes I think it is possible to taste when food has been cooked with patience and love versus when it has been rushed. Mum's cooking was the heartbeat that pulled us to sit down and eat together. She probably expected to see how well we had learned to cook later in life. I was quite looking forward to having her and Daddy eat many dinners with us as we grew older.

Once, we sat in the back of the car on our way to a local wildlife park with the family. Mum had filled a hamper with cooked tandoori-marinated chicken, often cooking sheesh kebabs to go with it. It left me with a mouth-watering taste whenever we ate grilled dishes. There were samosas mixed with pakoras; the salads sometimes had an Asian spice added to them; the yoghurt was mixed with mint sauce. All of this was jam packed into the food hamper. I used to catch a glimpse of my Dad's eye, where I was convinced that I could see how much he was enjoying the food Mum had made for him.

Mum loved family life and seeing everyone happy brought her joy and satisfaction. There were plenty of occasions to celebrate at home, be it for birthday parties or anniversaries. She loved preparing samosas and pakoras, or biryani. I could see from her smiling eyes how much she loved it when people ate her home cooked food. It made me happy because I believed people liked Mum's homemade food the same way I did. I loved seeing how she was quite modest when someone complimented her cooking. Relatives said the way she made mincemeat and macaroni was different to the taste they were used to. That dish was always finished with no leftovers. Friends would say Mum's Asian omelette was delicious and loved eating it with naan and yoghurt. She would bring in a plate piled high so that we could all share it. She spent hours cooking *khir* (rice pudding made with coconut milk, raisins, cardamom, pistachios, and toasted almonds), *gulab jamun* or sweet carrot halva. I know the other aunties did the same and their food tasted delicious too.

I appreciated how much Mum enjoyed her kitchen and her home. What was really lovely to see was that when Mum was cooking, her friends or the aunties would come and help or sit and chat with her. The kitchen was where all the conversations took place. It was like that back then, and it is like that now. The only difference is that I am doing the cooking. I know that when I try to make the same dishes today, it all takes that little bit longer, as I don't have the same patience that is required so I don't take for granted what I had back then, not for one minute.

Our birthday is in November, so kids who came to our party would usually get excited because they would receive an entire chocolate advent calendar, along with a goodie bag, to take home. Yes, these times were filled with happiness and joy.

Sometimes, I imagined Mum was seated in an empty chair with us at the dinner table, joining us from above, enjoying the mix of tastes that us children produced, encouraging us to keep going. Abbid loved Mum's cooking so much that I ended up recording him videos of how to make mince meat and potatoes with all the spices so that he could try to re-create the taste of Mum's food.

Home was where we would get our Mum hug until Daddy came home, and then we would get our hug from Daddy. We were a family of huggers. We talked about what was on our minds, listening to the advice Mum gave us. She called us Aishaneesa to speed up saying our names which we got used to. Ultimately, that's what I saw my parents as – advice givers with open ears to listen to us kids when they weren't busy working or cooking.

My life at home was full of love, warmth, stories, and laughter, which really mattered because that's where the bonding with my family took place. If I felt sick, I would look after myself by going to rest until I felt better. This was especially the case with monthly menstruation. I hated getting my period. In my experience, periods are one of the worst things that a woman experiences. (I don't have kids, but I've heard that childbirth is probably worse.) I certainly don't share the same wonderful feeling that Anne Frank described in her diary when she menstruated. I hated the stodgy feeling in my stomach as my uterus wall had a party every month with the heavy boom boom beat of eggs banging away to the boom boom beat in my ovaries. I hated the feeling of wearing a sanitary towel that felt like a brick. It wasn't my favourite part of pubescent life. The feeling of a mini volcano erupting inside was not anything that I looked forward to. However, it later turned out to be comforting knowing that women had sanitary towels with wings, yes, wings. This meant that no matter how wriggly or agitated my teenage self was from having my period, the wings kept all the blood inside my underwear.

I would wake up with a bellyache from my monthly period. Blob Blob. Is this what it was going to be like every month for the rest of my bleeding life? Whenever us girls had our periods, Daddy would carefully put a packet of sanitary towels into a brown paper bag at the shop to hide the item from our brothers at home. Menstruation was such a taboo topic in our household. We never talked about periods with anyone except Mum. She was always full of sympathy for us whenever we complained about having stomach and leg cramps.

I think the reason we never talked about periods at home was because it has to do with the body changing – which was embarrassing for us girls. As young children going through puberty, our parents could see how uncomfortable change was and left it to Mum to handle the girls' issues. They knew we felt sensitive each month and gave us the space we needed. It meant we could preserve our dignity without having to feel ashamed and awkward. I think overall not talking about this taboo topic meant I grew up into being quite a shy adult when it came to my body changing, but I am not upset with my parents because of it. I think they did the best they could, as I am sure any parent does. There is after all no guidebook on parenting.

When I had my monthly period, I got terrible stomach cramps around my belly that left me thinking about dying from the pain. Sometimes it was so bad that I used to think I was actually dying. Imagine dying from periods; what a waste of life. What a feeble way to go. I would find myself lying upstairs on Mum's side of the bed calling to her downstairs to come check up on me. I wanted her to see if I was alright so that I could display my agony to her.

"Mum! Mum! I've got a belly ache."

"I'll make you some hot milk with honey. Do you want cheese on toast with it?" She'd ask, being sympathetic. She would then bring me cheese on toast to go with a hot drink. It was in those moments I felt like I wasn't going to die after all.

I never quite understood how we could survive after bleeding continuously for so many days every single month. I started to wonder what boys went through in comparison. Having Mum around made me feel supported when I had my period; she made it all just about bearable.

Growing Up and Going Out

Then, boom by the age of fifteen, I felt like I had grown up with a mature enough attitude to conquer the world. A solid education filled with heaps of creative activity provided me with the feeling that I could achieve anything. After all, knowledge is power, is it not?

Mum made us home-made wax by mixing sugar and lemon, that we could use to wax off our Asian hair. We grew up waxing, not shaving, so after a while it didn't hurt at all. It meant the hair didn't grow back for about five weeks each time.

Both my parents had practically no hair on their legs which led me to wonder where we got so much hair from. In any case, we took the wax to the bathroom which had a strong pungent smell, working it into a soft state ready to apply to our legs. Then we would cut strips off of English magazine covers that had the perfect stiffness to act as a strip, applying them to the wax. Once the wax was stuck to the strip, I would gather some strength to rip it off. It felt great. It was almost painless provided you put enough wax on your leg but leaving enough time for it to stick to the magazine cover helped too. It left our legs super smooth for about five weeks.

Daddy realised, with four children, that we needed more space. So he had an extension built. To the right was the bedroom, to the left the study. That left enough space for a small en-suite in the middle. I loved sharing a room with Aneesa because we could chat away. We talked endlessly, laughing a lot too. As identical twins we knew each other like the back of our hands, completing each other's sentences, then moving on quickly to the next sentence. We were pretty lucky teenagers to have our own area to grow up in. I can't say I know why we were given this whole extra space to live in, but it enabled us to become a bit more independent from our brothers. We could also stay awake late, revising or studying without disturbing everyone else in the house. It didn't stop us talking though. That we did to no end. Maybe my parents needed space from us because we had so much energy to burn.

Once, I threw a deodorant can at Aneesa who swiftly moved out of the way. It impacted the wall, falling to the ground with a thud. Both of us immediately saw a hole where a small section had fallen out. It wouldn't have felt so bad were it not for the fact that a new extension had only been built a month earlier. Upon seeing the bit of newly formed wall crumble on the floor, we found ourselves cooperating quickly to patch up the mess. We filled in the hole with a mix of glue wedged with paper. We always found a way out of trouble. I don't even know if Mum noticed the covered-up hole. Maybe she did but chose to ignore it. The extension was a great space to be in where we had fun, although like most teenagers, we got on each other's nerves too. Thank goodness we lived in a detached house since it wasn't very quiet when we were in it.

We would be studying when one of us would suddenly say, "Stop. Tidy up!" This was because we shared a round table where one side was often a little messier than the other. We would stop right there to tidy up without any need for an explanation. We could have had separate desks but enjoyed sharing the same table to study on. It's not surprising that we were and still are close. These small things brought us closer together, and we never found ourselves having a conversation saying it was time we got separate desks.

We practiced the violin upstairs, occasionally getting a little clap for effort from our neighbours who either really enjoyed what they heard or were being polite, perhaps hoping we would get the point and stop. Having Aneesa there as my buddy was brilliant. There wasn't any activity that only one of us did. It probably created a little bit of healthy competition to practice together, or to see just how bad we were, and that we needed to practice more.

When Daddy drove us to family gatherings, we would usually fall asleep while trying not to vomit because we twins suffered from travel sickness. We often took two pairs of our clothes with us because we vomited so much. We did take travel sickness tablets but we could barely swallow them. When we felt sick, we would give Daddy a signal.

"Daddy, Daddy can you pull over now please?"

With that, he would smoothly pull over the car once he found a safe spot, which was luckily always just in time before we vomited. Then we would stand there trying to slowly get fresh air.

"Breathe in and out slowly" is what my family would say, which luckily worked most times.

When these moments of nausea happened, nobody could rush anything. Everyone would have to wait patiently until we were able to sit back in the car, usually with the window open so that we could continue our journey to wherever we were headed. Mum liked her perfumes so after a small nap during the car ride, we would be woken first by the smell of perfume that Mum would spray on herself in the car. This meant we were arriving soon. It was a gentle way to wake us up. She would say in Punjabi, "Batees, Aishaneesa, time to get ready." With that, we would wake up from a deep sleep to get ready for our visit. Mum would pass us the lipstick or hairbrush because after sleeping in the car, our long hair was usually ruffled, but by the time we stepped out of the car, it had been combed through again.

Being parents to four children was stressful. It reminded me of one time when we had all sat in the car ready to visit relatives in London. Daddy had been driving for about one mile, and suddenly Mum said she couldn't remember if she had turned off the gas cooker. In those moments, we all went quiet and held our breaths as Daddy had to find a spot to turn the car around and drive back home. This happened on more than one occasion, showing that our parents were only human, even though we saw them as people that we didn't expect would make mistakes.

Each perfume Mum used represented an occasion or memory - with a story attached that we would talk about after the event. We would say to each other, "do you remember when this or that happened?" knowing we were always there together as a family. She loved wearing her perfumes and jewellery whenever she went out. The make-up, perfumes and jewellery all sat gathering dust on the bedroom table once she wasn't there to use them. Aneesa and I didn't take the same pride in wearing them as Mum did. One of the strangest things I experience now is that I can sometimes smell the perfumes Mum wore around me even if there is no one in the same room as me. I don't know why the smell suddenly appears around me and can only guess she is around me somehow. It is also comforting and not scary at all; I feel happy in those moments. One of the exceptions was Mum's handbag that Aneesa had modernised into something she could use to make sure it didn't just sit in a cupboard gathering dust.

I recall a moment where we sat in the car after visiting one of our relatives. It had gotten late. We hadn't eaten much because the food was unfortunately too spicy for us to eat. Daddy was a little irritated because we were pleading with him to go to McDonalds. After he drove us there, I will never forget him saying he would have expected us to be able to eat spicy food by now, what with it being part of our culture. We should have been able to take the heat, literally. As he drove into the McDonalds car park, I looked to the car to our left recognising who was sitting in it. It was none other than our other cousins. Yes. They must have been thinking the same thing. We clocked onto each other being there. Nobody wound down the window to talk. We all looked across at each other with our eyes, quietly eating our burgers and fries. No words were exchanged. Each family understood that sometimes it's best not to say anything. Of course, we had a giggle afterwards on the drive home.

"See, Daddy, see! We weren't the only ones who found it too hot."

Mum made a point of making sure all four of her children cleaned the house, served guests with drinks, or set the table. She didn't differentiate between the girls or the boys. I found this interesting because when we were visiting others' families, I immediately noticed the difference. I think it gave us young girls the insight early on to see that it is possible to share tasks regardless of gender. It helped us form views that were not conventional at the time in some communities. Thank you, Daddy, for not blocking Mum's efforts at creating us as equals at home.

Traditional Clothes

One day, my older brother Abbid entered a competition with the local radio station, which he won. The prize was to be taken to dinner in a Rolls-Royce car. Daddy had to shut the shop early that day, which is something he never did, unless it was urgent or Christmas. That day, our parents were both beaming with smiles. Everyone was happy. We have beautiful memories of Mum dressing up in her shiny long silver traditional sari. Daddy looked great in his suit. Our Welsh neighbours, who were lovely to our family, came outside to see the Rolls Royce parked outside our driveway. We were all excited watching the car arrive to collect them. The driver opened the door for each of them. It felt special for everyone.

When we saw Mum in her silver Sari, she looked so elegant. We were impressed with how she put it on because we had mainly seen her wearing salwar kameezes. Ironing one wasn't a simple task either. We used to either lay out the material across the ironing board, or sometimes it was easier to iron it on the floor by putting it out on a sheet because there was more space. Mum would glide the iron across the material carefully with each stroke to avoid damaging it.

I wore salwar kameezes too. A salwaar kameez is a traditional outfit where the trouser part is wide at the waist but narrows to a cuffed bottom. A long ribbon is threaded around the wide waist bringing in the trouser part. A traditional tunic or top is worn with the trousers, hiding the ribbon. When I went to the bathroom, I felt like I was juggling how to gather up the top part into a ball, so it sat in a bundle in front of my stomach. The aim with the bottom trouser part was to avoid it falling to the ground. Anyway, I mastered how to keep it all compact, but it was never straight-forward. At least wearing trainers with a salwar kameez felt far more comfortable than wearing high heeled shoes.

Unlike Mum who managed to carry herself properly in the Sari, in comparison, one of my worst experiences of wearing Asian clothes was when I had to wear a lehenga that my parents had brought us. It didn't quite finish getting made the way it should have. A lehenga is a form of ankle-length skirt from the Indian subcontinent. It has beautiful embroidery on it which one would find at festivals or weddings. I found this two-piece item nice to wear since the pleated skirt part was easy to manage in the ladies' washroom, shall we say. Wearing a lehenga is quite an art. I think the ability to look natural in one, with the make-up and shoes, whilst being able to dance elegantly is something I admired in my cousins.

Lehengas can look rather extravagant. The colours look fabulous on anyone. The one I wore was lilac coloured. It was reminiscent of a chocolate bar called Milka which has a lilac-coloured cow for its branding. I asked Mum if she was sure about this purchase because it was very expensive. She loved how her daughters looked when we dressed up in traditional clothes. We loved seeing her happy. I was no fashionista, but I noticed that the material was heavily embroidered with the top slip part feeling a little tight. It could be closed by a zip at the back which would have been fine had the zip been attached to the material properly.

The day arrived when I had to put on the top part for the first time because we were going to a wedding. I needed help getting into it, so my siblings closed the back for me. My brothers were great in helping to get us girls ready that day. Unfortunately, before we left to get into the car, the zip ripped away from the material a little. The rip revealed the skin on my back. I tried to cover my exposed back with the long hanging dupatta across it. A dupatta is a length of material worn on the upper part of the outfit. It is arranged in two folds over the chest. It is then thrown back around the shoulders. That dupatta had in it thick, industrial staples that hadn't been taken out of the garment when it was being embroidered. I didn't notice the staples at the time because the dupatta was still being worked on. It had taken a little longer to prepare due to the extensive amount of embroidery. Clearly it wasn't quite finished because the staples were still in it! Let me be clear, when I say industrial staples, I mean that. They measured at approximately an inch long. They shouldn't have been there but, boy, they hurt my skin when they poked into it.

When the zip ripped, we noticed that the dupatta had staples in it. Being the Chaudhry's, we shifted from a tense moment of "Oh, no!" to bursting out laughing. The boys in my family found it hilarious. Mum was more concerned about whether I should get changed into something else or try to cover up the mishap. We opted for the latter.

My brothers were great. They kept sliding the heavy material whenever they walked past me to make sure it covered my back at the dinner. I tried hard not to move much at all throughout the entire evening. I had to keep apologising for not dancing on the dance floor. There was no way that this elegant lilac Milka cow was going to be able to pull it off.

When we got home, we all gave each other a smile which was a silent way of acknowledging how we all came together to help me out. I loved being in my family. We had lots of silly moments like that. We siblings were good at coming together to help each other out when needed. There was a strong bond there. With my brothers pulling together to help me out, I felt a bit like we were mini superheroes at home, only without the costumes.

My brothers' pitching in that day showed Mum how we

were willing to help each other, despite being boys and girls. There was a lot of unconditional love and joy that was felt in our family, and even though we argued a lot too - because which siblings don't? - she could see we were there for each other when it was important. I believe Mum imagined a future with not just us six, but as an expanded family one day, with herself in all of the family photos.

She would miss out on so many milestone events, be it to see some of her children get married, or to see how we helped each other later on in life at big important events. When those events did happen, our eyes filled with tears as we tried our best to be happy, knowing fully well that Mum was missing. So much joy and love was being built up over the years to be lost because she wasn't there to feel it.

Chapter 5
Turning Point

The Change in Life as we Knew it

Although Mum had grown up in Kuwait, she moved to the UK after getting married. Kuwait was a peaceful country until it suffered and parts of it were destroyed during the first Gulf War, when in August 1990, Iraq invaded it. I was around fifteen years old.

I watched my parents call the Red Cross regularly for any updates about Mum's family, who were living there. Nobody had heard from them for such a long time, so she was naturally very worried about them. News channels like CNN or Al Jazeera reported on the invasion, but she didn't hear directly from her family in Kuwait for months.

During this time, she travelled to Canada to be with her siblings, who were living there. I could only imagine what it must have felt like for her to not hear from her family in Kuwait. I realised how lucky I was to not have had to experience an actual war in England, where I just happened to be born. By the time the war was over, she heard from her family who had all survived.

That time in our lives was a pivotal turning point. When Mum got back from Canada, she didn't feel well, so she went to see the doctor. From that moment on, everything changed.

Sit back and listen, for I have a story to tell. I want to tell you how life was dramatically altered for our family. We all have dreams, don't we? We work hard, try to be happy, go out, control our health, do sports, hoping we can continue this pattern in our lives forever. But what one cannot do is have control over illness – not sickness, but illness. Usually, if you are sick, you go to the chemist after getting a prescription from your doctor. Taking medicine will eventually help you get better. This doesn't happen with illness, unfortunately. Much less with chronic illness.

In my story, chronic illness came in the form of a diagnosis called kidney failure. Humans usually have two kidneys but only need one to survive. We were taken aback to hear that both of Mum's kidneys weren't working. This meant she had to go on dialysis. It goes like this: One day, Mum went to her GP.

"You have a pain in your tummy… you're feeling tired a lot… you are leading an energetic life but getting exhausted, are you, Mrs. Chaudhry? Hmm, let's do some tests, shall we?"

Sometime later, after NHS tests, the answer was revealed.

"Sorry, Mrs. Chaudhry. You have kidney failure. It affects a third of Asians, who are prone to high blood pressure or diabetes. Do you have any history of this in your family, to your knowledge? No? We can't really understand why your kidneys aren't working. Although you only need one kidney to survive, both of yours aren't working. Mrs. Chaudhry, are you ok?"

We can spend a day or ten contemplating why her kidneys stopped working, but what good does that do? Upon listening to this news, Daddy cancelled any more work trips to Saudi Arabia for contract work so that he could stay by Mum's side.

Mum went quiet. She didn't complain. She asked questions. Aged thirty-nine, with four children, aged from 10 to 17, suddenly the future looked uncertain for Mrs. Annsa Chaudhry.

"What does this mean for my life? What about my family?"

In the back of her mind, Mum was thinking about her family. She didn't show any irritation or frustration but kept composed, asking what she could do about the fact that her kidneys didn't work.

"You should lead as normal a life as possible," said the doctor. "And can I get a kidney?" she asked.

"Mrs. Chaudhry, it isn't easy to find donors, unfortunately. You'll have to go on dialysis. A dialysis machine acts as replacement kidneys. It is a treatment where the machine filters waste products and fluids from your blood."

Dialysis was the only option for Mum to improve her current condition.

"In addition, you can join the list of people waiting for a kidney transplant. You need to decide if you want to be placed on the organ transplant list. An organ transplant isn't a cure for kidney failure. To be clear, it requires a fair amount of consideration, since this isn't a list that starts at number one. Nor does it mean you eventually get to the top of the list".

The consultant explained that kidney donors are matched by blood group and tissue type, so there is a better chance of finding a suitable match from a donor of the same ethnicity. With other organs, there is no requirement to match the tissue type.

Therefore, your ethnic background makes a big difference to your outlook if you have kidney failure. You read that right: there is no queue-jumping for kidney patients. Any chance of living a full and healthy life depends entirely on your heritage. The UK is a beautiful nation of multicultural ethnic communities, yet what is clear is that the largest number of people donating their organs mainly come from the white ethnic group.

The Hurdles Post Diagnosis

It was 1991. I was feeling bitter because it was at this moment that the consultant from the John Radcliffe Hospital in Oxford gave us worse news. Mum's blood group was B, rhesus negative, which was not very common. If her blood group was more common, like A or O, then her chances of finding a match would have been higher. This meant finding a match was going to be harder.

Mum also had several blood transfusions because of the loss of blood when dialysing or from the numerous operations that she had when her fistula[10] stopped working. Transfusions saved her life, but it meant her chances of a kidney transplant were reduced even further because each transfusion she received meant she developed antibodies. Each antibody in her body increased the chance of a donor kidney being rejected.

Unfortunately, you can't remove antibodies that develop after a blood transfusion. Once they develop, they are there to stay. They help you get better in the short term, but in the long term, they lead to rejection of the potential transplant.

I imagine it to be like being wrapped in a bubble wrap of antibodies that form in your body after a transfusion. Just when that perfect kidney comes along, it says, "Hello there, I am totally ready for this to help you live. I am that gift of life for you," only to be hit with a clear signal from the antibody saying: "Um, I don't think so. Sorry, we can see how it goes. Feel free to try to settle down but let me say now that I don't think you'll be staying too long." That is the kidney being rejected.

There were so many obstacles stacked up against Mum's chances to get a kidney: Her blood group was rare; the blood transfusions created antibodies; there were not enough donors anyway; the kidney had to preferably be from an Asian donor; Asians found the topic taboo. All of these factors reduced her chances of finding a kidney. How awful must it have felt to be told that because of those reasons your chances of successfully finding a kidney are extremely low. To be told this news by some consultant who showed no emotion whilst delivering the information to his patient must have been hard to hear. He was simply doing his job by asking if Mum wanted to go onto the transplant list, while telling her why her chances of finding a match were so low. He must have known that we were entering the realm of searching for the impossible. It didn't feel impossible to us, though, so we didn't act like we had been defeated. After all, Supermum had survived living in three different countries, she had survived a difficult pregnancy with twins, she had managed risky situations at the family shop, she had gotten through her own family living through a war, and she would manage this too. The reality was that we hadn't fully appreciated how difficult it was going to be to find Mum a match.

Mum faced many obstacles: She had a rare blood group; the organ she needed was one that required tissue typing to be checked; none of the family were a match when we tried to be living donors because of tissue typing not being good enough; and there were also many emergency blood transfusions. She faced one hurdle after another. Despite the extremely low chances of finding a donor kidney, Mum never lost hope; none of us did. In fact, our hope only grew stronger. Having hope helped us through it all. Our collective morale helped too. Morale gave us all emotional strength, which actually felt good. It was definitely going to be needed throughout the years.

Despite her illness, Mum still made the best of her life because she wanted to live it. She didn't let everyone see if she was feeling down. We knew she was often tired, but that was from the dialysis treatment or operations she had in the hospital.

We found out that there were already around 5,500 kidney patients waiting for a kidney. So what did we have to do to keep Mum alive so our family could all continue to live our happy lives? How could we make sure Mum would keep seeing us perform our songs in harmony, keep cheering us on in Judo competitions and watching us win, and teaching us about waxing? How long until our biggest worries would only be how to cover up a broken zipper at a party? Suddenly the level of worry had risen in terms of what to worry about. How hard was it going to really be to find her a kidney? What could I do to help? How did the UK handle organ donation?

Taboo Topics are Unspoken

We didn't want Mum to have to spend the rest of her life on dialysis because nobody knew how long her body would be able to take that treatment. It was, after all, only a lease for life. We all hoped so much that she would be able to manage dialysis without too many problems until a kidney was found for her. Luckily, dialysis did its job of keeping her alive. Thank goodness for that.

We'd say to the family, "come on, we can do it. Yes, we can. We can!" But, no, we couldn't do much because the fact was that not enough Asians carried a donor card. This was something we slowly realised was a massive problem for Mum.

There was a huge lack of awareness about the scarcity of organ donors amongst the ethnic communities. If anyone knew how hard it was to convey the message about carrying a donor card amongst the Asian community, surely, they would see how it felt like talking to a brick wall of people that sympathised but didn't want to be proactive or brave or donate after they died.

It was quite difficult, if not ironic, seeing how the Asian community we surrounded ourselves with reacted to Mum. They were very caring towards her being a woman in the community who needed help, but I slowly learned, it was a taboo topic. Respecting our elders was extremely important, meaning we knew it wasn't ok to raise the topic out of respect for them. We knew not to upset anyone who might feel uncomfortable. Praying for a kidney was easier than talking about how people could help.

Some people were against it because of what they understood

through their own educational learning or culture about the rules surrounding this topic. Burying the body whole was also important. People felt it took far too long to wait for tests to be done on a potential donor, which was problematic because it was important for burials to take place quickly after death.

We knew better than to enter into a dialogue with them. Therefore, we didn't force the topic on them. We didn't talk. If only they could see donation as permissible since it was seen by some religious scholars as an act of principle necessity. With that intention in mind, it could be considered a charitable act to help someone, rather than an unthinkable interference with someone who had died. But nobody talked about that. There was only deafening silence when it came to this topic.

Mum was the only person in our community who we knew needed a kidney. She practiced her faith in a quiet, subtle way. She did that without imposing her opinions on people; it was the same when it came to the topic of organ donation. She never imposed her wishes or hopes on people in our own community about how they could help. They could have helped by being a voice for her, by talking to each other, to their families and community about registering on the organ donor register. Sometimes it's easier when others speak for you. But that never happened.

The idea of being an organ donor wasn't considered wrong by Mum. So why was it so difficult to talk about it? The reason was because making people feel uncomfortable or awkward wasn't something we did. The result was that voices of patients desperate to get help were not heard. Conversations were not had. With so many strong voices of women in the community, there could have been fundraiser events as part of a function where the community attended. The women with strong voices could have spoken up in support of the need to talk about organ donation. I know events had been held where educated women were invited to give talks about certain topics. So why didn't anyone suggest speaking about that topic as a sign of support for Mum? I wish I had been brave enough to suggest it, but I wasn't. It meant I had not had a single discussion about the taboo topic with anyone about how they could support us and be a voice. I found that disappointing, but mostly sad.

It was hard knowing that a family like ours, with so much hope, was struggling to get talking. It felt so difficult to have a discussion with people on how to overcome the objections that they had formed because of their faith or culture. Unfortunately, ethnic minority communities, or communities with a strong religious emphasis, left people interpreting organ donation as something that interfered with their journey with God. It was often thought that if that was your fate, you shouldn't try to fight it. In other words, don't get in the way of what your fate in life was meant to be. Perhaps that made them feel less guilty about not being interested in being a voice for Mum – that is assuming they felt any guilt at all.

I had a small niggling feeling in the back of my mind that although people prayed for my Mum to get a kidney, they felt it shouldn't be at the sacrifice of a fellow member of the Asian community. Of course, I never found out if that was true.

Because no one could check with God directly if it would really be okay to not be buried whole, it was easier or more comfortable to not have to face the issue at all. This was what the thoughts in my head were telling me. I never verbalised this since it obviously couldn't be proven. My thoughts may have been completely wrong, but I didn't dare to bring up the topic. Furthermore, I didn't want to make anyone feel uncomfortable – just like Mum.

It's a bit like the phrase "Do what you want, but not under this roof," which equated to, "sure, I support you with your campaign for a kidney, but please make sure it doesn't come from our people".

I was left feeling deflated, even sad at times, because I

couldn't engage in discussions about what I thought people were thinking. Plus, their relationship with God wasn't something I was going to interfere with. My silence was simply out of respect for not being seen to challenge my elders. I should have been braver or more courageous. Perhaps if I had been, I would be sitting with my Mum here right now. Mum was subtle. She never wanted to upset anyone. She was a peaceful person who never complained or talked badly about people. She listened to conversations but with an open mind and without judgment. I learned from that as I tried to mirror Mum's behaviour when it came to manners and character. It was easy but also hard because I am naturally quite bold.

The Organ Donation Waiting Game

The best chance would have been from a family member who was a match. Our family was tested to see if we could be living donors for Mum but none of us matched. That was gutting. Living organ donation wasn't really very common at the time, so we didn't feel comfortable asking anyone. Nor did we expect someone living to step forward since we had been informed that kidney transplants were only thirty years old, which meant it wasn't clear how donation would impact a living donor who had their whole life ahead of them. It would have left us with a bad conscience because of the uncertainty of the donor's future.

Furthermore, being eligible for organ donation wasn't something that was easy either. An organ couldn't be taken from just anyone. In fact, any potential organ would have had to be tested at a hospital before being transplanted. Some people would not have been eligible to donate for a variety of reasons. For example, having a disease, being under eighteen, or having lived in the UK for less than twelve months would have made a donor ineligible.

However, if a dead person had been found to be eligible

to donate, which would result in being a match, then a race against time would have begun, since the organ would need to be donated within a certain number of hours after death. The patient would need to be brought to the organ quickly. Then some lucky person, a recipient, could receive their healthy organ. That lucky person could have been my Mum. Without her kidneys working though, she couldn't live without dialysis. Her chances of living a long, healthy life, were drastically reduced.

During the ten years Mum waited for a kidney, nobody we knew who might have been eligible to donate had died. She literally had to wait until someone who was already on the organ donor register died.

Even then, it would have still been necessary to get consent from the deceased's family. By then, emotions would be high. Would it not be better to know beforehand what the wishes of the person who died are, rather than leave it to the family to make that decision?

So for her, it really was a waiting game – waiting for the home telephone to ring or for the pager to beep, telling her someone who had died might be a match. For my family, it was a long, anxious wait.

Then there were times in Reading and Cambridge Hospitals where a donor was available, but the tissue typing was 75% against being a match for Mum, so it made no sense to go ahead.

Mum carried a pager around with her to get alerts from the transplant hospital in case there was a potential donor, but she only ever got an alert once. We wondered if the wait would be over. Daddy drove Mum from Reading to the John Radcliff Hospital with her overnight bags. They waited there patiently, along with another family. It turned out, the other patient, a young teenage boy was a better match. Mum didn't have a kidney transplant that night. I felt disheartened but kept myself hopeful that maybe next time there would be a kidney for her.

It didn't mean she wouldn't have stood a chance if she had received a kidney from a white donor, since most donations actually come from people from a white background. It simply meant a better match would have come from someone from the same ethnic background as her. But the chances of that happening were so low.

When Mum and Daddy got home, they told us how it was extremely tense while they waited. The flow of information being given to them was good, so they were kept up to date, but it wasn't meant to be for Mum this time. Mum had said how it was a blessing that anybody got the kidney; she didn't want to be in front of anyone. She wanted everyone who needed it to get one. It was gutting for her. Clearly, it meant the wait wasn't over. Would it ever be over? We still had hope that the call would come, but the call never came again. I didn't realise back then how little her chances were of getting another call. That was quite worrying, leaving me feeling stressed, wondering all the time how she was doing since Mum had her highs and lows with dialysis.

Once, when we visited Mum at the Hospital, we saw a Black woman who had received a transplant. Her two young children, aged around eight to ten-years-old, sat by her bedside. It felt fantastic to see. You couldn't feel anything but happiness for that family, knowing that their lives would be changed forever. We knew about Mum's kidney failure when our younger brother was only eleven. How great it would have been for her children to see their mother live longer. Hopefully, she would have had more freedom to do what she wanted in her life.

People say it must have been hard whenever I met someone who was a transplant recipient, since Mum, who we saw spend so much time in the hospital for the next ten years of her life, didn't get hers. I didn't know how to answer this so simply, but my heart only feels love for that family. They deserve a happy life like anyone else. A single person deciding to donate is all it takes to make a difference for someone and their family. That is why I was happy for this Black woman who got hers. How grateful we must be that people are selfless enough to be organ donors. Just take a moment to think about that.

Sometimes, when we visited Mum whilst she was dialysing, it was like going into a static but highly intense time warp. The patients were sitting on their chairs whilst their lives passed by. Nurses monitored them, acting quickly if something wasn't right. Our family was in a constant state of heightened tension. We would ask Mum how the fellow patients were doing since it was them who she spent her time with when she had her treatment. She would say a little sadly, that even though they have husbands or wives or partners, they felt very alone. No one visited them. One of these patients was another Asian woman.

It is true that the stigma attached to having an illness can lead to patients not telling anyone that they are being treated or need life-saving treatment. Nobody would know that their outlook in life or the length of it could be shortened.

The amount of stigma that surrounded this taboo topic was not only amongst the ethnic minority communities, but amongst the public. There had been several cases of mistrust amongst the medical profession resulting from hospital scandals.

I had read reports about South Asian countries where living donation was more common than donation after death. They saw living donation as a way to support the family financially. One reason was that these cultures are very family-oriented.

Even though humans are born with two kidneys, they only need one to function. Arguments amongst the medical profession and ethicists had dealt with the idea that people should be allowed to sell one of those organs to help them and their families financially. On the other hand, there had been cases of trafficking of human organs, raising concerns about the misuse of organs.[11] Not all countries had regulatory frameworks, thus in some places there was an increased risk that the donor could be exploited or harmed physically.

During the ten years, a couple of uncles in Reading and Pakistan had explored the idea of searching for a donor in Pakistan, India, and Egypt. The first person wanted to sell his organ. His blood was collected at the Airport and tested at a private Harley Street Clinic in London but wasn't a match since Mum's blood group was not a common one. It was B, rhesus negative.

The second person didn't have a close enough tissue type match, and it wasn't worth moving forward. These people were from abroad. The consultant in Reading told Daddy that he could not approve of it because even if Mum went abroad and had the donation there, he would not be allowed to manage her aftercare when she returned. The NHS didn't support this route for Mum due to the reasons above. There were too many uncertainties for the donor, including whether they had actually agreed to donate or if they had been pressured into it. Even the level of care the donor would receive during or after the donation wasn't clear. Not to sound barbaric, but nobody knew enough about how this could work for anyone involved. Furthermore, there was no guarantee of how the aftercare would have been for Mum, after a transplant from a donor whose medical history the doctors weren't familiar with.

Once, Daddy had visited a kidney transplant patient with my uncle, but upon visiting, he found out her kidney had been rejected after transplant. He said she was really suffering, and it scared him and uncle about how bad things turn when something doesn't go as well as expected.

Daddy explained to us that despite looking into the option

of finding a donor from abroad, moving forward with finding a donor from outside of Europe was never going to be a viable option for Mum. It was hard to hear, but it was absolutely understandable because of the legal and practical obstacles. We had to accept what we had been told. I felt demoralised knowing that in another country far away where Mum had been born, there could have been a match for her. Because that pool of donors happened to be in a country which wasn't in Europe and had different infrastructure to where we had grown up in the UK, Mum was not going to benefit from that pool. On the one hand, I felt sad because a potential path had been found, but deep inside I was relieved that neither the donor nor Mum's well-being were put at risk. Simply imagining a bad outcome because of the risks made me feel nervous and nauseous.

Nobody would have known when Mum left Pakistan and Kuwait to move to the UK that she would one day be waiting for a kidney from a small pool of Asian donors. I made a mental note to myself to bear that in mind when choosing where in the world to live.

When Family Matters Become Public

I was fifteen; Mum thirty-nine. She told us what the doctor had said (blah blah blah blah blah). "Yes, Mum. What, both your kidneys don't work?" We listened avidly to what she had to say. It was like Cinderella being told that not only can you not go to the ball each year anymore, but that you must stay in and sweep floors forever. We were crushed out of this world as the earth moved away from below our feet. Mum fought to survive. With the news that she would be dialysing, we quickly understood that she had been granted a lease for life. Little did we know it was an extension for a limited period of only a further ten years. Even towards the end, she continued to protect her children. She said, Inshallah, God willing, I will be okay. She never gave me the feeling that the situation was desperate, protecting her children from the imminent death that awaited her.

One day, the headmaster of our school asked me to talk to Daddy. Given there were only five other Asian kids in our school of 1500 children, perhaps the headmaster was impressed at the large number of activities us twins were taking part in. Growing up did have growing pains, but it balanced out with the fun we had at school. Every time there was something to take part in, we were there. It was a great way to get to know kids in the years above or below. Being the sparkly, bright-as-light-without-a-sigh-in-sight twins, nobody noticed that we were a bit low about the news of our Mum, which was probably because we hadn't mentioned what was going on to anyone. We didn't say anything because it was a family matter. No one needed to know what was going on at home.

The headmaster wanted to ask Daddy to be a governor. Daddy was reluctant to take on such a role, explaining that he would find it difficult to commit time to the school because he was running a shop. He said he needed to be available in case Mum needed him. What we were facing were serious family matters.

My Dad telling the headmaster about Mum's illness was the first time the idea of death hit me deeply. Without having experienced it before, I found myself spending time thinking life was going to be over for all of us soon. I couldn't stop thinking about death. I had this warped unrealistic idea that even at the age of fifteen, my life was going to be over quickly. I couldn't imagine living into my adult life. Those were irrational thoughts, but I found myself thinking about thoughts like that. We were facing some serious times ahead. I had to get into the right frame of mind after the initial shock of hearing about Mum's illness. I panicked, thinking to myself, oh no, does this mean that we've been sprung? Do we have to act all sad now, because that wasn't how we wanted to act or feel. Nobody knew Mum had an illness, but now everyone did, or at least to me, it felt like they did.

Of course, we had told our close friends, but the idea of everyone knowing made me feel uncomfortable. So I went to school as usual, except I felt like the whole school, including all the teachers, were watching me. Did this mean I would have to explain to everyone what dialysis was? Would I have to tell everyone what it meant to need an organ transplant? Perhaps I should have asked for the school to hold an assembly explaining what it all meant, because maybe then, when everyone asked, "How's Mum?" we wouldn't have to say "Fine," or "On and off."

The fact sheet we could have provided would have said it all. It might also have said that Annsa is a dialysis patient who will have to spend large amounts of time on a machine, but also in hospital because she will be prone to infections. If she has operations, she may have to have blood transfusions which are only given when too much blood is lost. Losing blood often happens with haemodialysis. Her fistula is connected to a vein and artery so it could seep, which means it needs to be kept clean. That area will be fragile and shouldn't get infected. A catheter will be attached to the front of her stomach, so she won't be able to sleep on it anymore. That it will need to be kept dry when showering to reduce the risk of infection. It's also important to stay away from patients who have dialysis if you aren't well because they have a weaker immune system, which means it'll take longer to recover when they get sick. All these things sound so dramatic, but that is because they are.

I was sixteen and in the final years of school. I had finished giving a presentation on why there should be trees in the sixth form area because then we could all get more oxygen. I argued why we should try to save trees because of their capacity to help the environment from the oxygen they provide; thereby improving air quality. Perhaps instead I should have told everyone about why I thought it was important to carry a donor card at that ripe age of sixteen, the age of curiosity, rebellion, standing up for our rights; or getting our voice heard.

In hindsight, it would have been a good idea to talk although at the time we wouldn't have known what to say because we didn't have the tools to help us say what we wanted people to hear. Mum didn't tell us how she felt either and we were too young to know how to explain it all in a meaningful way.

In the early years, dialysis went more smoothly. There were good days, absolutely normal days when all went well and Mum carried on with life as normally as possible. That's definitely how it was for Mum in the earlier years when Daddy took her out for her birthday or took the family out to see a theatre show. It's important to note that there were good days. Over time, we would often come home to find that the day hadn't gone smoothly at all for Mum.

Dialysis left her with cramps in her lower legs or around her stomach. When Mum's skin got dry or itchy, she applied E45 cream to it, but it didn't seem to help enough to soothe her from the itching, so it would bleed. The skin would recover in time, but it was hard watching her have the urge to scratch while trying to resist it. Occasionally on peritoneal dialysis, it led to an infection called peritonitis, which can be life-threatening. She did recover from those infections but it usually involved an emergency visit to hospital.

For haemodialysis, some parts around the area of her entry points for her fistula were so fragile that it caused the skin to seep a little with blood. Those times made my stomach turn. We would constantly be on the phone keeping Daddy informed if Mum required emergency treatment. All of us children would keep in contact with each other about what was happening next with Mum. When the ambulance came, whoever was home would wait and watch Mum get collected after the doctor had signalled that she had to go in for treatment or help. Sometimes, it meant a trip to the hospital nearby in Reading. If it was serious, as was often the case, she would be admitted to the John Radcliffe or Churchill Hospital in Oxford, or the Addenbrooke Hospital in Cambridge where there were specialists who could help with her fistula. Yes, my heart raced as did all of ours, and yes, she always made it home thanks to the amazing work of the medical staff. Daddy drove there after work to see her, or we would take our study notes and spend the day there if possible.

Mum was a proud woman who made a conscious effort to dress elegantly. She put make-up on to feel good. We did the same to keep up our family spirits but watching her suffer meant there was a constant feeling of anguish in my gut. The worry grew stronger, lasting a little bit longer over time. It became almost permanent. The feeling that she was invincible also became imprinted in our minds. We had subconsciously expected that she was going to be in our lives forever. What a paradox! Her mind or willpower never weakened though. That remained strong. So did we.

I think explaining all of this to my school friends in detail would have made it harder, not only for me but for them too. Since everyone has had a Mum, or Dad, or guardian, or caretaker, they could easily relate to how real it all was, making it a bit too close to home. It's easier not to have to think about difficult things happening at home. It was far better not to show how bad or worried I felt because that was easier than having to answer questions about what was going on with Mum. I remember a very close friend at school once commenting on how little time we had to drink water during the school day. She said that I of all people should have drunk more given that my mother was waiting for a transplant. I knew she was right, but I also acknowledged to myself in that moment, that I was ignoring the seriousness of Mum's situation. To face the reality and accept the difficulty of it, made me feel scared to death. I also think not being asked if I needed support at school was fine for me at the time. In an indirect way, it felt like the teachers looked out for us anyway. So I chose to bury the severity of it all and instead to do the British thing and keep calm and carry on. That was the easier option. I gave myself hope because by ignoring it, I believed all would be fine.

Given that we were bubbly twins, I didn't want to make others feel sad or sorry for us, but maybe then the message would have gotten across quicker to everyone around me. Maybe it would have encouraged people to ask us about how to get the donor card or how to get onto the organ donor register. I would have said you can get the card from your local doctor's surgery, at the hospital, or at the pharmacy. Instead, I focused on getting the grades I needed to pass school exams. It was a wasted opportunity to spread the word.

Visiting Kuwait

The Gulf War had impacted Mum's family hard until it finally ended in 1991, when I was sixteen. Even though Mum would have loved to visit her family in Kuwait, she couldn't since she was clearly not fit to travel and because she had to undergo dialysis. Instead, in 1992, Aneesa and I were sent to represent our family on behalf of Mum who couldn't go herself.

I don't know why my parents chose this point in time. I wasn't even sure about whether to be excited or scared about going, not least because our relatives had lived through a war. I couldn't even begin to imagine what that must have been like. We were about to set foot where our relatives had lived in a war zone. Having grown up in the UK, we had never been anywhere near a war so we couldn't relate to their experience at all. Perhaps I was scared because it meant spending time in an unfamiliar land where people spoke Arabic, not English; perhaps it was because I knew they had been hurt by the impact of the war.

British culture was so different to Asian and Arab culture. I could see it at home when Mum communicated with her friends. Although we grew up enjoying a mixed cultural household, my lived experience was completely different to where I was going to venture. I grew up in a home where English, Punjabi, Urdu, or Arabic were spoken. For me, family life was full of British baked beans, enjoying a cup of tea and a biscuit, and Asian biryani being served with Arabian delights like baklava. I loved the mix of all of this. The mix of intercultural communities is what made my life so special. It was all around me when I grew up.

The volume of a room full of people talking loudly created a vibrant atmosphere of everyone happily mingling. They were cooking in the kitchen, playing cards, sitting outside together in large groups chatting away creating a hive of activity. The sounds I heard of people speaking, the smells of food, the continuous laughter was good for my heart. Laughter is the key to happiness. Such a rich tapestry of cultures was wonderful to grow up around.

What was it going to feel like visiting relatives in an Arab country whose lives were so culturally different to mine? I saw with my own eyes how it was from the moment we arrived. It was hard hearing what they went through to survive the Gulf War. We were well looked after by everyone, feeling immense love from the family, but I found it incredibly hard to hear first-hand stories from them about what they had experienced.

One aunty told us that women had to dress up to look ugly so that they didn't get taken advantage of by men out there, because assaults on women were not unheard of. I didn't want to hear it, but had to listen, because it had happened. They wanted to tell us how it was for them. I couldn't do anything about what they told us. I could only be sorry. We were shown windows that were still completely sealed to keep out the fumes from chemicals let off outside. I wondered how it must have felt to be stuck inside during the hot weather if they wanted fresh air.

We were driven around Kuwait by relatives who showed us where Mum had gone to school. I imagined her playing when she was a little girl. They also showed us the roads that were lined with palm trees, explaining how that's where people had been buried after the war. It was heartening to see that Mum's family was safe, but it was awful to see the effects of the invasion of Kuwait. One uncle had asked us to pass a book to my mother. When I looked inside it, there were gratuitous photographs showing graphic images of how the people had been wrongly treated by others. Images are etched in my mind of the torture endured. I wish I could forget those images, but can't, which is surprising given that I only flicked through the book.

As a sixteen-year-old teenager, I found it hard to swallow that people could be so cruel to others. I didn't want to show the book to my Mum, since I wasn't comfortable sharing the horrific images with her. She had been through a lot, so I didn't want to stress her out. But her family had been through a terrible experience too, clearly wanting her to have the book. The book we were given remained in one of Mum's drawers in her room. I imagine she had looked through it, but we never talked about it with her.

Mum's family was living a completely different life culturally than ours since we were living in the Western world, whereas they were living in the Arab world. The smell in the air was completely different to where I had grown up in England. The air in the UK could be so cold it went to your bones. In contrast, the air in Kuwait was dry. When I drank the Kuwaiti water, it had a smoothness to it. I watched my uncles chop all the herbs using traditional blades, instead of using a blender or mixer with a plug. That looked quite cool. The fridge had been packed full to keep everyone fed with healthy fruit and vegetables. It was such a small country but the generosity of the people in it was enormous.

I went upstairs to the roof briefly to collect some washing that had been hung out to dry. That's when it hit me. I am talking about the fifty-degree Celsius heat. I had never felt that sort of heat before or seen how quickly socks could dry outside in that temperature.

Once, we went to the British Embassy with an Aunty who worked there. One of her colleagues who had caught sight of Aneesa and I started talking to her. He said he had cousins in the UK in Leicester who needed wives. We looked at each other thinking "No way!" How dare he? Luckily, our aunty wasn't having any of it either.

What a relief. We joked with her afterwards, asking, "How much did he offer for us? How many camels plus the dowry?"

I am glad we were born in the UK, since us girls had freedom in our lives that we would not necessarily have had if we had grown up where our parents were born and raised. When we were at weddings, us twins would happily go around saying hello to the aunties, (you called everyone aunty whether they were related to you or not) only to find ourselves being stared at by women we didn't know.

They would summon us over with their index finger, looking at us closely. They asked us if we were engaged to be married yet. I think the WAYMY question usually got directed to the guys more from what I remember. Why Aren't You Married Yet? When we told Mum what the aunty said, she would smile without saying much. She never really probed us which I quite liked. I think Mum wanted us to be free in the world, to be independent strong women. I am very grateful to her for that.

Chapter 6
Keeping Calm and Carrying on Despite It All

Driving Miss Aisha

At the age of seventeen, I took driving lessons. Daddy organised for us to have lessons with one of his customers, who was a relaxed, cool Rastafarian man who wore a large Rastafarian hat. I thought Daddy was cool for letting us have driving lessons with him. Whenever we had gone to our music lessons before then, it had been Mum who took us in the car. Soon, we could do it ourselves. Admittedly it took me five times longer than Aneesa to pass my test, but I got there in the end. Yes, I took five driving tests.

I failed the first test for driving at forty miles per hour in fourth gear around a round-about. When I got home Mum said, "Don't worry *Beti*. Next time. You'll pass next time." Then, to cheer me up, she would cook up sweetbread which worked a wonder. Sweetbread was like French toast. It was basically a slice of white bread that had been dipped into a mixture of eggs, milk, and sugar. It tasted even better when it was slightly overcooked leaving the edges all chewy. Mum knew it was one of my favourite dishes.

The second time apparently, I didn't stop in time at a stop sign. I thought the Examiner purposely pulled up the handbrake before the car even got to the stop sign. The third time it was foggy, so they almost cancelled the test, but we went ahead. As I drove the car out of the forecourt, I was hit with the feeling that the Examiner didn't really want to be out driving with anyone at all. I think he wanted to cut the test short, which he did. I was irritated because it felt like he had failed me before I had even started. The fourth time I was possibly a little too enthusiastic. I drove a little too fast, scraping my instructor's car against a pavement edge. I took my instructor with me on the fifth test. Finally, I passed. The moral of the story is not to give up. When I got home, Mum gave me the biggest proud Mum hug ever. She said, "Finally, my *Beti*, you did it. Wait till Daddy gets home. He will be very happy."

He was happy I passed but it might have been because I had cost him over £1000 in driving lessons. After I passed my test, I loved driving Mum around to show her that all my efforts had paid off. She loved it too, because with the fistula on her fore-arm it became difficult for her to drive the car because there was a risk her arm would bleed. Those big achievements followed by the recognition and hugs from Mum put such a huge smile on my face. The unconditional love for all the effort meant so much to me.

I miss not being able to share magical moments with Mum anymore; where we were both filled with excitement after achieving a goal. Daddy has been brilliant to share our joy with instead. It lifts us all up when we have something to celebrate. I had to learn that there was no point living in sadness and regret. I also learned it was impossible to fill Mum's shoes. Not that there was any expectation, but she gave us so much love and did it really well.

Living on Dialysis

For the first six years, Mum was on peritoneal dialysis. She spent twelve hours a night attached by her tummy to a tube, which was connected to the machine. Of course, people can have a comfortable time dialysing. It isn't difficult for everyone, but over time, it can be a big strain on the life of a patient. That's how it was for Mum. She was mentally strong;

her willpower impressive, but ten years of dialysis took its toll on her physically.

There was no black-and-white picture of life on dialysis that could be drawn. Nobody's experience was going to be the same as anyone else's. One simple hindrance was that with the catheter attached to Mum's stomach, she was unable to sleep on it anymore. She had cramps in her stomach and legs, which meant we spent endless amounts of time massaging her to provide her with some relief. She had to monitor her water intake daily and the sorts of food she could eat. Dialysis took place four to five times a week. It was rather draining on Mum's time, often leaving her with less energy in the later years. Sometimes, she would come home feeling good. Other times, she was completely shattered. During those days, she would go straight to bed, getting up only later after resting.

We regularly received deliveries of about fifty large Baxter boxes at the door with bags that were full of saline liquid, which is required for dialysing. These boxes were moved into the house monthly, just as they were moved out of the house once empty. We all lined up to bring them inside. They took up the entire entrance floor area all the way to the top of the wall. Sometimes we came home to find them all outside, behind the gate, where they had been left by the company delivering them. The drivers always helped to put the boxes where we asked them to, and they were considerate of the fact that they were dealing with patients undergoing life-saving treatments. Not all delivery people are compassionate, but the ones who came to our door from Baxter were. We would then have to move them in slowly together. This took a while because they were heavy from the saline in each bag. This went on every month for six years until Mum had to switch to haemodialysis, which she couldn't do at home.

Daddy did his best to make the most of life with the family too. After having closed the shop for the day on a Saturday, he would collect Mum from haemodialysis. They would sit in the car together, enjoying eating a samosa together. I found that romantic; it reminded me that they really did love each other very much by taking that time out to sit in each other's company. It made me appreciate the sort of relationship that they had where Daddy spent time with Mum.

I looked back at how turbulent that time in my life was; the memories flooded back about how it felt to be in my family when I was younger. The variety of things we had done from going to see musicals with Mum, the events Daddy took her to that were with the Asian community, her children making her proud from all the concerts we sang at or judo competitions we won, they all made Mum happy. They made us all happy. I reflected on what a wonderful, vibrant life we had. We didn't sit and wallow in our sorrows. There was no point because it didn't help, and in all honesty, there wasn't much to complain about anyway. We were blessed to be a close family that talked to each other and turned up when it was important. When it came down to it, time was what mattered. Being around the family and doing things to grow and keep us busy made us happy. Of course, I still loved eating those samosas whenever I visited Daddy in my adult years. He worked so hard at the shop to provide for us all. When Mum felt fit enough, we would go out to visit relatives or her friends. Doing this lifted her spirits. It was fun, too.

Mum had to go to the hospital often because sometimes her fistula wasn't working or she got an infection, so we all spent many summers and Christmases at the hospital visiting her. The staff were nice enough to let Aneesa and I sing Christmas carols to the patients.

We went Christmas carol singing to raise money for the dialysis unit, which was fun every time. Singing usually put a smile on people's faces. One year, we were singing Christmas carols outside people's front doors. We rang one doorbell thinking the family wasn't home because nobody opened up. We started to walk away. Just then we could hear a woman calling for us to come back. She had her new-born baby with her. That was a magical moment with the mum listening to us while her baby slept peacefully. We sang Silent Night extra quietly to her, watching her holding her baby that night. We told Mum all the stories when she was in the hospital about what we did, telling her who we saw when we were out. She loved listening because when we arrived, after settling down by her side, she would ask us to tell her how our day was. Then we would start talking and not stop until she got tired of us chatting away. I knew she was tired when her breathing became slower, or if she wanted to move from sitting upright to lying down. I can imagine that with all the chatting we did, we wore Mum out. Sometimes we just sat quietly by her side, reading through our study notes while she was resting. It made me feel good keeping her company; knowing she was not alone for longer than she had to be. That was when we left her alone to get some rest.

For quite a few years, when Mum ended up having to stay in the hospital over Christmas, Daddy would collect the turkey to cook at home. We marinated it the night before in Tandoori paste mixed with plain yoghurt and mixed spices. We would then place it in the oven early in the morning, ready to take it to Mum once it was ready. We knew she couldn't eat much, especially when she was in the hospital, because she was usually sick if she was in there, but that way she could celebrate Christmas with us. We only took a small plate in for her because she couldn't eat much anyway, but we still went in to be with her. It was important to us to be together as a family. Taking in some of the Christmas dinner had to be done because it brought the family together. We all felt better for it.

The staff at the hospital were really understanding towards

us, having gotten used to seeing the Chaudhry family there over the years. It made us feel happy that we could be together like all families, trying to still celebrate events together despite Mum's condition. We did our best to make the most of these because they put a smile on her face. Seeing her smile when she was down made it all worth it. Any excuse to celebrate was fun. So, fun is what we had. Lots of it.

Thank goodness Mum loved to celebrate events and occasions with her family. She wore her good clothes and jewellery to look and feel great. The vibrant colours of the salwaar kameezes were worn with pride whenever we went out, and she definitely made an effort regardless of how she was doing with dialysis. She often positioned her dupatta carefully around her shoulders and neck making sure it didn't make contact with her fistula when it was on her neck, to prevent any risk of infection.

Dividing up her clothes to store in our cupboards at home after she passed away was incredibly hard to do. Aneesa and I didn't wear those clothes everyday like Mum did. Taking them out of her wardrobes and putting them into our closets was more for memories. I rarely felt the same enjoyment when I wore them because I was doing it to represent Mum, when it was her that should have been wearing them. I would go on to hear aunties mention decades later, that they recognised something of Mum's that we were wearing; perhaps a piece of clothing or jewellery. Knowing they recognized something of hers was bittersweet. Then, we would get emotional together and talk briefly about her before putting a smile on our faces.

Daddy was quite romantic too. When it was Mum's birthday, he usually had something lined up to surprise her with. It would usually start with him going off to work early, like he did every day. Then, when we were all awake, we would go to see Mum who would tell us what gift he had left under her pillow. It was usually a small piece of jewellery. Then he would take her out to watch a show combined with a meal.

He would take Mum to London to watch Asian Melas. A Mela is a meeting which is usually a large gathering for people who enjoy bhangra music. All types of Asians, be they Sikh, Hindu or Muslim get together to enjoy the rich vibrant sounds for the whole night. It is a big performance where Asian musicians would perform with dancers looking colourful in their outfits. Instruments would be played including a sitar and tabla. Of course, tasty Asian food would be consumed. When my parents went to these events, which unfortunately wasn't often enough, they returned home happy, looking culturally nourished. They would talk about who they saw that evening, who was on stage, what food was eaten and who they bumped into.

On the other hand, we kids much preferred going to see musicals at the West End theatres in London. I don't know where this started from, but Daddy had once taken Mum to watch the musical Cats by Andrew Lloyd Webber. She said it was amazing because of the music and costumes. We were intrigued. I wondered if she might have liked watching performers because we had seen photos of her when she was a student in Kuwait performing traditional Indian Kathak dance. The emphasis was on using the eyes, hands, and feet to express oneself, with photos showing Mum doing exactly that. I asked her about those photos, listening to her describe what she was doing with this form of dancing. There was even a cool video of her belly dancing with some of my aunts. They were all enjoying themselves while dancing away at one of the many family gatherings.

Sometimes, I think Mum was more open-minded than we were when it came to us girls growing up. If there was a programme on television with doctors on it talking about a woman's body, we said,

"Mum, that's rude!"

She would say, "Then, watch it upstairs. It's educational! You might learn something."

I am sure she only approved because it was doctors giving out the information. One of my funniest recollections was when we went shopping with Mum. Having tried on some tight-fitting T-shirts, I said to Mum that they felt too tight around the chest area, "Mum, the tops are too tight. They show my shape too much" to which she replied, "Good, there's nothing wrong with it." I was quite surprised but wondered why it bothered me about how the shape of my cleavage could be seen from the T-Shirt I had on, when it didn't seem to bother Mum the same way. These were the small ways she helped us teenage girls feel confident in our bodies. That made me feel comfortable, so I didn't worry so much.

One of my favourite memories with Mum was of her taking her daughters to a restaurant for lunch after we passed our A-level exams. It was one of the few times she took only the two of us twins out without our brothers. The lunch felt special. I felt really grown up. We were all happy spending time watching Mum be so proud of us both. Usually, we went out to restaurants for meals all together, but here it was just the girls. Mum sat opposite us; her brown eyes beaming with pride. We had fun that day, smiling at our success and laughing when we told stories about how stressful it had been studying during the last two years. I felt relieved that we had made it, but it was clearly a sign that we would soon be leaving home to go to university.

I remember hearing parents talk about having only eighteen summers with their children before they left home to forge their own journeys. I did the same when I went to university, and I was looking forward so much to keeping Mum up to date with what was going on in life. As a child, I was happy to have the chance to fly the family nest and get some independence, but I naively thought Mum would be there for me to share those stories with when I was in my thirties or forties. I didn't appreciate how limited my time was going to be. In one way, that meant I lived and acted as if life with Mum was going to go on forever; on the other hand, it was naive thinking. Perhaps I would have spent more time at home, but I know Mum got so much joy from her children doing things in our lives. It lifted her up, and we shared so many stories with her about what we were getting up to. It separated us from the routine life she had to lead on dialysis. I think she was happy we had freedom. In fact, I am sure it made her happy.

Adulthood Beckons

Time passed quickly. I had turned eighteen with a tonne of memories combined with life-shaping experiences behind me from my time at home. Aneesa and I went off to university for three years, followed by law school. University was the start of many firsts. It was the first time anyone from our family had moved away from home to study. I made new friends, learned how to survive without my twin and spent a huge amount of time figuring out how to enjoy my new freedom next to studying.

My family drove me by car from Reading to Essex. It was a long journey of about ninety miles. University was an exciting time for me and I was curious to see how long I could go until my family visited again. The quick fix of eating pasta in my first semester wore off quickly. In the end, it tasted pretty bland. This meant it was time for Mum and Daddy to visit since I craved Pakistani chicken with coriander the way Mum made it.

First, there was the announcement of a visit. Daddy had to get up early to open the shop around 6:30 am so it was a tiring trip for him. Given Mum had to dialyse overnight, the visit usually started in the afternoon. By the time they arrived everyone felt nourished with love where we all connected again.

Daddy brought a supply of long-life food or energy drinks for me that I kept in my room for a rainy day; Mum showed me again how to make Pakistani chicken so it tasted like hers. I was well fed and happy. Then there was the sadness after they had gone. My friends at university were so supportive. I would meet them after a visit from my parents and talk about what we did. We would have a cup of tea and try to find something to laugh about before the evening ended. It was the same for them when their families left to go home. We would meet and talk and try not to be too sad. Living away from home was an important learning curve. Coping on my own was something I had never done, so it was good for me to grow myself a little too.

My time at university from the ages of eighteen to twenty-one was enlightening. I was far too sensible, but honestly speaking, a fair amount of time was spent checking with my family on how Mum was doing since she was in and out of hospital so much during that time. I had the best support from the housemates who by now knew my Mum's situation. They were great during these tense times. I never knew if I would wake up thinking I better get on the next train because things had gotten a little complicated at home. Usually my family told me not to worry and to stay at university, so I trusted them and only travelled when it was absolutely necessary.

Looking back, I can say on a positive note that I realised I loved to have fun and make people laugh despite the difficult times. I also found out that dancing was a good outlet. I had never really tried to dance until I went to university and had so much fun when I danced the night away. I saw how my parents did their best to try to let me have a normal life at university. I appreciate that now, but somehow wish I had learned how not to worry so much. Unfortunately, it was hard not to, given how uncertain Mum's condition was.

Mum spent time in a total of eight different hospitals,

including the John Radcliff Hospital in Oxford, the Churchill Hospital in Oxford, Addenbrooke Hospital in Cambridge, the Royal Berkshire Hospital in Reading, the Dialysis Unit in Reading, Dellwood Hospital in Reading, Wokingham Hospital in Wokingham, The Battle Hospital in Reading, ending at The Middlesex Hospital in London. Her life was spent continually battling with the symptoms and side effects of organ failure. The numerous complicated operations she had were usually as a result of infections or from needing a fistula to dialyse. She had a remarkable amount of patience. As they say, all good things come to those who wait. It's only because of the hard work of the medical teams who helped treat her successfully so many times that she came home each time. To them I am extremely grateful.

I was lucky enough to have access to a phone in my room at university where I could listen to voice messages. I am glad the university let me have this machine in my room because it kept me connected to my family and what was happening with Mum. No one else I knew had one. I often rushed home after a lecture to listen to the voicemail messages telling me what the current news of the day about Mum was. I could only receive calls or listen to messages on the answering machine but couldn't make calls from it. Where was Mum? How was she doing? How long had she been in the Hospital? What were the doctors going to do? Was she going to need an operation? Was her fistula still working? Did she have an infection? Did she have cramps? Did she dialyse properly? How long were we going to have to wait to hear some good news?

I immersed myself as fully as I could at university so when I got back to my room from lectures or tutorials, or from studying at the library, I listened to the answering machine messages. There were so many of them, where each time I was left some piece of information by my family before I anxiously picked up the phone from the call box inside the halls of residence to try to find out what was going on.

Beep.

Aneesa: Mum's in hospital as you know. Everything is ok. They are just going to check her arm to make sure it is ok, but it means they have to feed her through tubes, which means putting a tube down her nose for about a week to ten days, which she is not happy about. Daddy is quietly stressing out.

Beep.

Aneesa: Update. Mum's had the tube put down her nose which has caused discomfort because it's rubbing on her nose where the bone is, so it's bleeding. Daddy seems a bit down. Call Mum at the hospital as it'll make her happy.

Beep.

Daddy: Good news, your Mum's home so hopefully things will be better by tomorrow.

Beep.

Mum: Salaam Alaikum *Beti*. How are you? Ok, I want to ask your opinion about which subjects your brother should take for his A-levels. Have a think and I'll call you back. Ok, take care. I love you.

Beep.

Mum: Oh, you're not home. Wherever you are, have a nice time. I will try to catch you again later. Take care of yourself.

Beep.

Mum: Hello *Beti*, Salaam Alaikum. I thought I'd talk to you but you're not home. Wherever you are, have a nice time and I'll talk to you later. I love you.

Beep.

Mum: Hello *Beti*, Salaam Alaikum. I am at Churchill hospital in the Oxford Transplant unit because my fistula isn't working. Hope to talk to you again soon. I love you.

Beep.

Aneesa: I phoned Mum, she sounded alright. There was a bit of a problem putting the needles in for dialysis, but they managed to do it. She should be home soon.

Beep.

Aneesa: Hello Aisha, Mum had the operation, and it went ok. Beep.

Daddy: Salaam Alaikum Aisha, it's your Daddy. Mum is still at Oxford Transplant unit after the operation. You can give your sister a call and she will give you a full brief on it.

Beep.

Mum: How are you, *Beti*, Salaam Alaikum. I am just calling to find out how your exam went. I love you.

Beep.

Mum: Salaam Alaikum *Beti*. I am sure you are in but you're asleep. I am waiting for the transport to come and take me to Dellwood Hospital for dialysis but they are late so I thought I would try you but you're not in. Guess what, I got a lovely present for Valentine's Day. I'll let you know. Love you.

Beep.

Daddy: Your Mum called you this morning and you didn't call back. She's not upset. Maybe if you give her a call, she'll feel more cheerful.

Beep.

Aneesa: I just wanted to know how you are and to see if you had the number for the transplant unit because Mum went in today, but I don't know the number. Don't forget to call her yourself to see how she is because her operation is tomorrow.

Beep.

Daddy: Aisha, it's me. Just call home when you get in. Beep.

Mum: Salaam Alaikum *Beti*. How are you? We haven't talked in days. I've got a letter for you from the Bar Council for Law School so give me a call and I'll tell you what it says. I love you.

Beep

Daddy: It's your Daddy. I just want to know how you are. That's all. Beep.

Aneesa: Mum's going to Oxford Transplant Hospital tomorrow morning. Not sure if you are going there.
Beep.
Aneesa: Mum's back as they decided not to operate and will wait a few weeks to see if things improve with the fistula.

It was during my third year at university, when I was twenty-one, that I went to Portugal through the Erasmus programme offered to countries in the European Union. I studied law there for a semester with five other students. It was while I was there that Aneesa wrote me a long letter letting me know that I had gotten a place at law school to further my legal training in London.

I could hear the excitement in Mum's voice when she left messages on the answering machine, telling me I should give her a ring. I could hear how proud she was in her voice. I talked to her on the phone afterwards, she told me how happy she was that I got a place. It meant that after coming back from Portugal, I wouldn't be moving back home. I think it was a bittersweet feeling for my parents, who loved having us around them, but on the other hand, I am glad that they were completely open-minded about letting us live away from home to follow our dreams.

Chapter 7
Serious and Surreal

From Bad to Worse

Mum wanted to get out to enjoy life despite her dependence on dialysis. Six years after treatment began, a trip to Munich, Germany had been arranged. It was a carefully planned trip where she took her Baxter boxes of saline with her. There must have been a dialysis centre that had space for her to dialyse during her stay.

To say it was an absolute disaster would be an understatement. She had to fly back urgently because she had an infection called peritonitis. Upon landing, she was transported straight to the hospital in an ambulance. Daddy telephoned us all, to tell us what was going on. We were all worried sick about her. It left me wondering if she would recover at all since peritonitis can be life-threatening. Mum recovered, but it resulted in her never being able to have peritoneal dialysis again. Nor could she dialyse from her stomach anymore. That moment was really scary and worrying for Mum and for us all. We didn't expect to hear that her life-line to the dialysis she was having was no longer possible. I didn't appreciate that there was the risk she would lose access to dialysing from her stomach. That made me feel sick to my stomach and I wanted to know what it meant for Mum. Once again, we had to wait for her and Daddy to explain what it meant for her. This was a déjà vu moment. Only six years earlier, we had heard Mum tell us what the consultant said when her kidneys stopped working. Here we were again, wondering how they were going to help to keep Mum alive.

What now? The consultant explained her options. "Mrs.

Chaudhry, you have to have a different form of dialysis called haemodialysis."

I originally thought Mum was better off on this dialysis because her body wasn't wasting away the same way it seemed to be when she was on peritoneal dialysis, but maybe I was wrong. She appeared to be building strength, but it meant she could no longer dialyse at home. Her freedom had been restricted. She had to travel to the dialysis unit in Reading, Berkshire, to have her haemodialysis. What an eye-opener that was! The risk of getting an infection was higher; her body was deteriorating faster. Perhaps it wasn't a better form of dialysis for her after all, but she really had no other choice. I felt nervous about how long she would be able to have this new form of dialysis. Had I started a timer, I would never have imagined that her time would run out only 4 years later.

This new form of haemodialysis resulted in a fistula being inserted into her arm which unfortunately, after some time, stopped working properly. Once an entry point on one part of the body stops working, a new place has to be found to be able to continue treatment. This eventually led to her having dialysis from the side of her neck. It was distressing for her; we could all see that. Yet she still made efforts to look her best whenever we went out somewhere. The fistula was protruding out from the side of her neck, wrapped up very carefully so that it remained clean.

The level of extra hygiene at home was necessary because if Mum wasn't careful, she was at risk of infection. It was incredibly hard to see my Mum who took so much pride in her appearance, having to adapt to those tubes coming out of the side of her neck. How she slept without being afraid it would get squashed when she leaned on it, I will never know. I just know she was brave, like all the other patients going through the same treatment.

One by one, her options of where to have dialysis on her

body were running out. The entry point for this fistula was keeping her alive. That's what mattered to all of us, most of all to Mum. Her body looked quite different by now when compared to the start of her journey on dialysis. It had been through so much.

Her dialysis entry points moved from her stomach area to her arm, then from her arm to her neck leaving scars each time. Each scar showed how strong her body had been to go through so much, leaving a visible mark each time to remind her of what it was capable of being put through to keep her alive. It makes one stop to think about how much a patient goes through when they are having dialysis. Sure, you can live a normal life on dialysis, but with the number of operations Mum had, you can see why it was important to have hope that she would get a kidney one day. The grass always seems greener on the other side, doesn't it?

There were, of course, a variety of difficult situations that could occur, depending on the impact dialysis had on a patient. Things could get very difficult. In fact, things got very difficult for her. Things got shocking. Shocking was seeing a fistula protruding out of a vein and artery on one side of your mother's neck. There was a powerful flow in the fistula. Once, it got disconnected, which was not meant to happen. It resulted in a strong fountain of blood that spurted out. It was messy to say the least. We stood watching, frozen, while three or four nurses jumped into action to contain the situation. The nurses acted fast while battling to keep the tubes connected to Mum's neck so that the whole system kept working like it was meant to. I admired them for their fast reactions; they acted quickly yet remained calm. They weren't panicking, but I could see how these emergencies created so many feelings of tension, ranging from surrealness and distress to eventual relief, not only for Mum, but for each of us. The nurses focused on their job until they got things back under control. The reality was that the loss of excessive blood meant another blood transfusion. Merely thinking about what I saw back then makes me feel dizzy.

Daddy witnessed this happen at the Churchill Hospital too when the nurses had attached Mum to the machine and the force of the blood going into the machine was so strong that the tubes flung out and blood was going everywhere. Daddy said the nurses apologised and gave him a cup of tea and sandwich afterwards explaining how the machine must have had a fault because it didn't usually do that.

Throughout the whole period, I had never seen a body decline so much one day, only to build strength the next. It showed me what an amazing piece of work the human body was. It could be fragile one moment, healing itself the next.

Just as those shocking moments happened a few too many times, we all managed to recover from the heightened whirlwind of distress every single time. More often than not, Mum wasn't ok. Neither were we, but she never complained or gave up hope of getting that kidney. Her willpower was exceptional. That's what people said to me at her funeral.

She never stopped believing. None of us did. She would say, "This is just something that happened," not blaming anyone. The hope was passed on to each of us over the ten years. I say this because I honestly don't know how we coped with watching her deteriorate in her physique without it. My eyes filled with tears instantly when I could see what was happening to her. It made me feel so helpless since she was the one going through so much in order to survive. She couldn't say she didn't feel like dialysing because then she wouldn't have survived. We couldn't exactly rotate her suffering between us, even for a day, which left me feeling sad, that it was her suffering every time. That didn't seem fair to me.

It was particularly hard when Mum came home, telling us how someone had died. Each time that happened, I realised how desperate her situation was. There was one young man who was in his early twenties who had died. There was also an Asian woman, like Mum, who had died. Mum's dialysis schedule meant she saw those patients often so when their time came, and she heard they didn't survive, it really hit her hard. This harsh reality that dialysis could only go on for so long made me feel sick to the stomach. We didn't talk about it much when someone lost their life in the world Mum was living in. She was in her own thoughts, worrying, but not saying much. We were tired too, knowing that, despite her strong faith, we couldn't rely on prayers alone. We needed some sort of action, but we couldn't see a way forward.

Graduation, Law School & Moving Away

I came back from Portugal and started law school in London, which wasn't easy for me. Mum faced many more emergency situations that led to her fistula being operated on, resulting in it being moved to a new location on her body. I had a great study group, but my mind was constantly distracted from wondering how things were at home. I am lucky my parents let me have my independence, enabling me to pave my way while carving out my own life. Yet I still found myself spending large amounts of time travelling from wherever I was, to see Mum when she wasn't doing well.

Once I completed the legal training, my proud parents saw me being called to the Bar of England and Wales as a barrister, dressed in a wig and gown. Being called to the Bar at Middle Temple Inn in London was one of the best memories for my parents. It was different from them coming to watch me take part in a judo competition or perform at a music concert. I felt proud that I had managed to finish the course in the time frame of one year. Not everyone does, even without all of the anxieties going on in the background. My goal was simply to finish the course I started, not to mention that it was expensive. I was glad that Mum was there to see me at the ceremony, along with Daddy of course. There was one photo that was taken, where Mum was stroking my face while she congratulated me. I cherished this photo because it made me see how my parents were when they were most proud. I have looked many times at a photo of me standing outside Middle Temple Inn, where I was called to the Bar of England and Wales. I knew that being there made their day.

Perhaps qualifying as a lawyer was the ultimate achievement of pride for my British Asian parents. I should mention that my parents didn't tell me to study law. I chose it because of the idea that someone else could be a voice for people who didn't have their own when it mattered. I couldn't think of too much else that I did academically where they were that proud, but celebrating the success was important, so we celebrated with a family meal. We talked, we laughed, and we had dessert. We celebrated like any normal family. It felt great to be together again.

I had found training to be a barrister at Bar school hard. The whole experience was very stressful for me. I was continually under pressure, trying to cram in everything while at the same time being distracted by what was happening at home. Living on edge with such intensity about Mum's health was incredibly hard, yet I had become used to the constant state of uncertainty. It became a part of my daily life.

I progressed in my own career, completing most of the practical legal training for my pupillage at a barristers' set of chambers[12] in London. I was trying to figure out my way in life, doing my best to gain some professional career experience along the way. I learned from my time in chambers in London that I would have to go to the law courts all over the country with my pupil master or pupil mistress.

In London, my pupil mistress would see me dressed in my black suit, white shirt, and tights, and say how my attire was appropriate. She also said I should wear the same outfit for my time spent training with her. I was irritated because I would have preferred to have some flexibility or wear trousers, which were more comfortable, but most women didn't wear trousers then. Not only that, but the table I sat at where I did my training was an old wooden table that ruined my tights every time they got caught on the rough wood. I constantly carried a spare pair of tights with me everywhere for that reason. I was far too polite to complain or say anything, which didn't make it easier. I had to get up early in the day to travel to a court somewhere in the country for the hearing. This annoyed me to no end because I learned from my pupil master or mistress what the day in the life of a barrister usually required. It was a ridiculous routine which included things like the law clerk sending instructions late in the day for a case that had to be heard the next day. Little time was left for planning the case. One had to travel early in the morning to a court, arriving there by 9 a.m., ready to represent the client.

I watched my pupil mistress quickly switch shoes to her small pumps to run in. Smart thinking. I then had to run with her to keep up. It was fun at the beginning, until it most certainly wasn't. Honestly, it wore me out. I didn't enjoy any of it.

Plus, the topics of family law or divorce law were far too emotional for me. I realised they were absolutely the wrong subject area to be working in, given all that was going on at home with Mum. Those cases were full of broken hearts, leaving my heart broken too. I saw how badly people who once loved each other hated each other when the gap between them was too wide to allow any kindness in. I was continually worrying about the weaker party, which if my pupil mistress was not representing them, felt uncomfortable to me. Although I knew this from my training, it felt like, with everything going on with Mum, I was managing enough stressful emotions. It drained me, depleting me of my usual energy which I was trying to keep for more important things.

I realised working in chambers felt alien to me, leaving me feeling awkward and uncomfortable. I didn't fit in. I pondered whether it was meant for me to spend my life working as a barrister. I already knew it was not. This didn't seem to be the future where I imagined myself being happy. I told that to Mum when she asked me how it was going. When I told Mum about how stressful it all felt, she often said, "Try to be happy, *Beti*." I think she could see I wasn't happy at all during my time training in London. On the one hand, I was happy that Mum and Daddy were proud of us for finishing university and going to law school. Thank goodness they could both celebrate seeing that, but inside I didn't feel confident in myself about doing the work of a lawyer. It was exceptionally hard and didn't appeal to me as something I could become passionate about – and I was ok with that. I just needed to figure out what to do instead.

I didn't expect my parents to tell me the answer to that either. I had to figure it out on my own. I would tell Mum I didn't know what to do for my job, and she would say, "I don't know *Beti*". It was my journey to go on and find out for myself.

I needed to explore something different. Despite all the great friendships that had been formed with friends that felt like my second family, it was time to try something else. I needed to discover what I wanted in a career in the hope that it might help me pave a path to happiness in the working world, without shattering my parents' joy. It turned out that I could complete some of my legal training abroad, which felt great. I wanted to feel excited again about the topics that I had studied, thinking time abroad could help.

Having spent time in Portugal during university, I decided to dip my toes into gaining working experience in another

European country. I talked to Mum about my thoughts, explaining to her that I felt like finishing my legal training abroad could be worth exploring. I wanted to know what the culture was like in another European country. I decided on Germany to see how different it was from Portugal.

Mum accepted what I was telling her. By October 2000, I was heading to Germany. I wanted to see how I coped outside of my comfort zone. Besides, I could easily hop on a flight to London Heathrow, if need be, couldn't I? It was only a two-hour flight after all. Who knew I would have to do that not too long afterwards. I didn't even take the full twenty kilos of luggage with me, but I took my excited little self out there, ready for some new experiences.

The interesting thing was that my parents didn't stop me. I think by this point in life, it was clear that nothing was going to stop me from living a life for myself. I felt the antagonism of wanting to be at home, yet I also felt compelled to step outside of my comfort zone. I had to see what it was like. Daddy had always said that if we had the chance to experience working abroad, we should do it. I recalled him saying how he had done it, so we should try to. I had been abroad to Portugal with the Erasmus program and then did some training in Germany, so it felt like I had to try out working abroad. So I did. Besides, I was regularly in touch with my family about Mum's condition. Thank goodness the mobile phone was invented by then. I am grateful my parents didn't sit me down to have a big talk, telling me that I shouldn't go. I was growing up, forging new paths for myself in life, not knowing where it would take me. The path to my future was also not back home in Reading, so I wasn't close by to home like I used to be.

In Germany, everything was very different from what I was used to. It felt far less formal, but things seemed more process-driven than in England. People started work at 7:30 a.m. I saw one lawyer wearing white socks with a dark suit and dark shoes at court which made me giggle. I was surprised the white socks didn't seem to be an issue for them. I cast my mind back to standing in front of my pupil mistress, waiting for her approval for what I was wearing. The white socks would have been an absolute 'no no' in chambers in the UK. The workers seemed far more relaxed in their attire for court. I felt more comfortable overall, telling Mum how much more relaxed everything felt. I think she was happy that I was happier. I described to her how things felt easier going than in London where I had been trained; that even though you sat with lawyers, you didn't have to wear the wig and gown the whole time. I should have felt proud wearing one, which I mainly did when I dined with fellow barristers, but I didn't ever practice in court so I managed to avoid having to wear one. It felt so pretentious. It was my choice to study the subject, and my choice to not practice. Mum was mainly relieved that I was less worried and was even smiling a little about the idea that I could use my skills outside of a courtroom. Luckily, I had managed to find a way to do that later in life.

During all this stress, Aneesa had the brilliant idea that we should celebrate our 25th birthdays. This was a great idea since Mum was turning fifty that year too. We thought celebrating this big number would be a great occasion for a party. It was almost like the party of all parties for us twins. My brothers were coming to the party too because we tried to do things with all of the family whenever we had the chance to. We invited about 100 friends, which included friends of the family. We told Mum to invite some of her district nurses, who spent years of their lives looking after her. They came all the way from Reading to London to be there. They loved it. We did too. It was fun, fabulous, and glamorous. Best of all, Mum was looking well – the best I had seen her look in ages. My memories from that day will stay in my mind as happy memories forever.

Aneesa rented a room with a stage, decorating it in all areas. People were happy to bring a dish to share. We sang some duets. Aneesa sang more songs than me since she was learning how to sing jazz at the time.

Lots of guests knew the party had been organised to boost Mum's morale since she had been going through a tough time lately. That evening, she was beaming, happy, smiling, and laughing. We could all see it. She was feeling good. One of my friends said she dressed rather elegantly, looking like a princess at a party that had been organised for her. She said it in a heartfelt way because she knew what Mum meant to me. In some ways, that was true; it was our party, but it really had boosted Mum's morale.

Everyone could see it. Guests went to talk to her, whom she hadn't seen in years, which she loved. The photos still made me smile long after the event, because I could see how much fun we had in between the seriousness of Mum's situation. She had even prepared a handwritten speech, but we only found it in her handbag a few months later when we were going through her things.

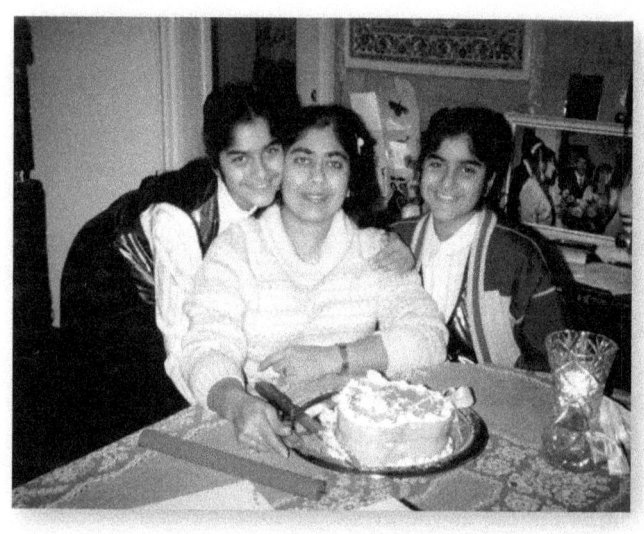

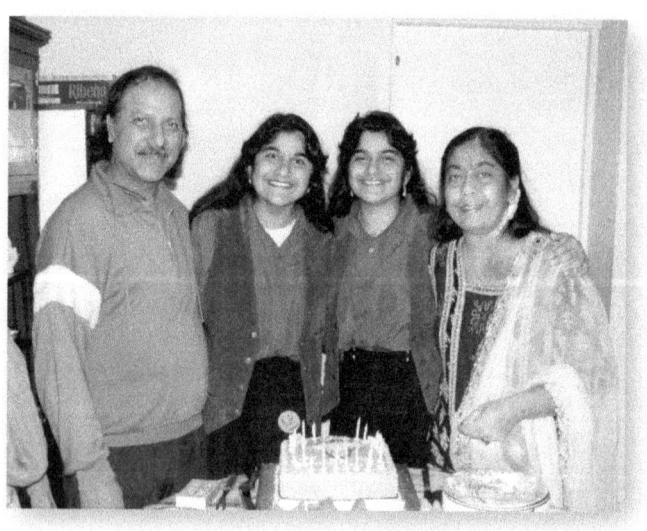

Chapter 8
Unknown Territory

Learning to Come to Terms with Dying

I learned about diverse cultures from growing up in a mixed-cultural home. I learned how to become a grown-up woman in a British Asian household in the UK. It was great. I wish, however, that I had been better prepared for what was to come because time with Mum was running out.

People often ask the question, "What do you want in life?" Of course, it is to be happy, right? But have you ever stopped to think about the single thing that you cannot control? No matter how much money you might have, regardless of who you know or where your background stems from, did it dawn on you one day when you woke up that perhaps you would be stripped of your good health?

Thank goodness for health, because when it suffers, it affects everyone you care about, be they friends or family. We saw how lucky Mum was to have the option to dialyse because, without knowing when a kidney would ever become available, it's what kept her alive. It's as simple as that.

As a set of four children, the second half of her ten years saw us watch her health decline. She had the willpower to get through her illness, but the impact of dialysis was taking its toll on her body, raising endless uncertainties. I had so many questions. Was I going to see how she handled getting all her children through university? Who would I complain to about women's health matters like fibroids or what the right age was to have a mammogram when I got older? Was I ever going to watch Mum go through menopause to learn from her experiences? Would she be around when I got older so that

I could share mine? I had assumed Mum would be there for her daughter so that I could ask her things as I grew up into adult life.

Situation Critical

It was 4 December 2000. Mum had turned fifty. We had been celebrating our 25th birthday with her only two weeks earlier. I was already back in Germany and happened to be skiing with friends in Austria for a long weekend. On 9 December, I sat in the car to head back to Germany. I contemplated how lovely it would be to take Mum and Daddy to the Alps to see the mountains and snow one day. I am certain they hadn't experienced the beautiful views from a hut in the Alps that you could get to by cable car. I thought it would be nice to show them how I skied. That was wishful thinking to say the least and couldn't have been further from ever becoming reality. There was no roaming mobile phone service in Austria, so I hadn't received the messages while I was in Austria. I only heard them once I was back in Germany. I could see that I had received a tonne of voicemails from Aneesa over the last couple of days.

What I heard was distressing. It was awful. I found it hard to listen to while travelling in a car between countries without an airport nearby. Aneesa had left me messages saying that Mum was at the Royal Berkshire Hospital in Reading with pneumonia. She was terribly sick. To make things even more complicated, she appeared to have a problem with one of her heart valves, which wasn't working properly. It was called a mitral-valve deficiency. The nurses said that giving her this medication had to work because they didn't really see what other options there would be within the Royal Berkshire hospital in Reading to help her heart.

Aneesa left a message for me saying that they were calling relatives because Mum was getting worse. I don't know how she caught pneumonia but I do know that if your immune system is weak, which happens when people are near you who have a cold or are full of germs because they are sick, then you are more likely to get sick because your immune system is already low. You can't easily fight off whatever bug or virus a healthy person has.

I had never ever heard anyone say, "They are calling the relatives," but somehow, I knew it meant that things couldn't be more serious than right now. It's as if they were telling the relatives to come so that they could say their goodbyes. What did I do? I got home, packed my luggage, and was ready to board the first flight to the UK. I had knots in my stomach, wondering if I would make it or if I was going to get there too late.

The hospital told Mum that she would have to take some seriously strong medication to try to get better. She was given lots of medication, but it wasn't really helping. The doctors told us that if it didn't work, they couldn't confirm what the options for her would be. We only knew that if she didn't get better, then they may not be able to help her in Reading, since the issue with her heart required people who were experienced with the heart. We were all in limbo, wondering what was needed for her to improve.

Five weeks later, it was quite clear that the medication wasn't working. The problem that resulted was that one of her heart valves needed to be looked at by a heart hospital. It meant that she had to be taken to the Battle Hospital in Wokingham, Berkshire, which was a bit further away than where we lived. It wasn't far like the transplant hospitals at Oxford or Cambridge, where numerous operations had been performed on her to insert her fistulas for dialysis. The staff at the Battle hospital concluded they didn't have the right specialist to be able to help her, so it was decided that she should be taken to London to the Middlesex hospital for surgery on her heart valve.

For our family, we didn't really know what this meant for us. After all these years spent waiting for a kidney without success, we were now facing a critical situation with Mum. We had reached a point where we didn't know what anything meant anymore. We were only familiar with kidney issues with dialysis. We knew that she needed a kidney transplant, but none of us were familiar with the heart organ or the complications of her valve not working.

We were naturally concerned about her heart not working properly because, in the end, any of your organs can underperform, but if your heart isn't working, then you're in trouble because that's the main organ that keeps you going, isn't it? Was it because of her pneumonia? Was it because of all the years of dialysis? Was it because of some other reason? We didn't have the answers to any of the questions.

Mum was transported in an ambulance to a hospital in London. Understanding hospital spaces or bed allocation in London for a family like ours, who came from Reading, was quite a big adjustment. The ambulance driver took Mum to London. Aneesa was in the ambulance with her. The driver got to London only to be told on his radio that the bed was no longer available. They asked Aneesa to sign a consent form to have Mum driven back to Reading, but she didn't feel comfortable doing that. Neither did the paramedic. He said she was too weak.

The driver then took her to another hospital, which was St. Mary's Hospital in Paddington, London. She stayed there overnight, even dialysing because she needed it urgently. That whole time was traumatic for us all. It was incredibly frustrating for us to see, given she was in a critical condition anyway. It was distressing knowing that they had put Mum in her vulnerable, fragile state into an ambulance, only to pass her around hospitals when she was at her weakest. Finally, she was admitted to the Middlesex Hospital in London to the heart ward. Everything felt cold. The staff seemed to be on a different level. Where was the empathy, compassion, care, or kindness we had grown used to from the Royal Berkshire hospital staff?

It felt foreign being there because it was. The staff were talking to her as if she were new to being a patient in a hospital. One nurse was particularly rude to her when she explained what Mum could or couldn't do regarding her water intake, so Mum, in her calm voice, explained that she knew what her water intake should be. She told them she had been dialysing for ten years. When you are struggling to breathe anyway, you don't want to have to use your energy to calm a nurse down who has a bad temper with an attitude that stinks. The nurse quickly changed her tone with Mum after finally reading her medical notes. She became kinder and respectful and visibly more sympathetic. She was probably stressed from her day, and now had a new patient to look after. I understood later how hard those nurses were working, but at the time our stress and expectation that Mum should be treated better, usurped any consideration that the staff were overworked.

Firstly, she was told it wasn't clear when she would have her heart operation. Then, they told her she was not really a patient of theirs. They said they were only babysitting her since she was really a kidney dialysis patient. Except she never had dialysis there. Not once. She had been sent to London specifically because she needed a heart operation by a heart specialist. Why did they make her feel unwelcome when the doctors had decided it was where she absolutely needed to be? She didn't get in the ambulance and drive herself there on her own, did she? It was clear she needed the operation, so she was going to have to wait patiently until a slot became available since she was too weak to be taken back to Reading now that she had been admitted. Mum didn't have the energy to react.

She couldn't breathe properly anyway due to her failing heart. Talk about pushing you when you're already down on the ground. It was not what I expected to see from people in the caring profession. That was not what we were expecting, not when we had seen how well she had been cared for in Reading.

Mum didn't even dialyse once at that hospital while she was there. She was there for her heart, with no efforts being made to dialyse her. I couldn't fathom this approach. Having dialysed for ten years, suddenly she wasn't dialysing every other day like she had been doing in Reading. Nobody told us why. Was it a budget issue that meant she couldn't use one of their machines because she was being admitted from outside London? They made the point of telling us she was being "babysat?" in the heart ward, as if to suggest she shouldn't have expected to receive dialysis there. Was her heart situation so dire that they didn't want to dialyse her, or worse still, that she couldn't be dialysed anymore? She needed her heart operated on urgently, yet she wasn't getting any dialysis in the meantime. This made me feel sick to my stomach.

As a family, we were all frustrated. We were angry. Getting some answers to our questions or explanations would have helped us understand what was going on, but we got no answers. From here on, I knew things were bad. My thoughts were telling me that the care she received from the medical staff in Reading was so much better than how it felt to me like she was being cared for at this hospital. I was probably being unreasonable in my thinking, but I felt like I had a right to be. Since it was my Mum who was in their hands now, I obviously wanted to see things being done properly. But I couldn't judge if they were or not. Instead, my thoughts wreaked havoc in my mind.

As I looked around, taking in this new environment of working professionals, they seemed distracted – disinterested, even. I recall feeling livid that the care wasn't there. We were clearly in unknown territory, which wasn't doing Mum any good. It wasn't doing her any good at all. She was vulnerable, weak, and probably scared. My family were scared too, feeling uncertain about everything. Uncomfortable at not being able to ask questions like we had been used to doing in Reading. I felt bitterness towards the staff at the Middlesex, who in my subjective view hadn't done the best job that they should have done for any patient, for my mother! I was, of course, comparing them to the staff at the Royal Berkshire Hospital in Reading, where Mum spent much of her time being a dialysis patient. This singular subjective view was only formed because of the experiences we had at this hospital in London. We were relying on them to save Mum's life, and desperate that it would go well.

My thoughts were probably highly irrational, but I asked myself how it could be that when they got it right for her for all these years, over a span of ten years, then how is it that in two short weeks it seemed to be going very wrong? When I say they got it right, I am talking about how they treated her when she was a patient there. Watching her progressively deteriorate because her heart wasn't working was so painful.

I asked myself, who knew what the staff were really going through or what pressure they were under? But you know what? I honestly didn't care. I didn't. I just wanted Mum to be looked after properly and couldn't see that she was. She was clearly in a dire situation, so for us, it was reasonable to expect that this place would have been able to look after her, to help her, to fix her heart. Little did we realise how slim her chances of coming home were. We desperately wanted her to come home again, but that was wishful thinking.

I believed Mum knew in this hospital that there was less optimism for her all around. There was less certainty for her about what lay ahead for her future. It was during this time that she prayed more than ever, while we were all waiting with her to see what would happen next. We let her talk into a cassette recorder to say whatever she wanted to. We wanted to hear her thoughts, so to pass time, we recorded her voice. I listen to her words on the cassette tape even today because they are a reminder of my strong memories of Mum. She shared her words of wisdom, her dreams, and her wishes. What a gift it is to still have this recording of her voice.

I still have the cassette tape where her weak voice could be heard; how her breaths were stagnating. Because her heart wasn't working properly. She was incredibly tired, but she was leaving us her wise words of wisdom as a mother, a wife, a daughter, and friend. Maybe she knew something; maybe she knew her life was in danger. Perhaps she knew in the back of her mind that she would not make it home. Here is some of what she said.

Mum's Recorded Words On Cassette

"I love you. I love all of you and inshallah Allah (God) will keep all of us safe and I will come home after a successful operation. Allah help me. Make me fit and let me have a successful operation so that I can go home to my children. I love my husband, my children and everyone including my family in Kuwait. Always have faith in God because you can depend on God. Inshallah He will help us.

Everything will be alright because I believe in one God, and He is my Allah. God gave us everything, He never let us down. This is just something that happened. God knows my wishes. Inshallah once I am fit, I can go to Mecca.

Of course, I want to see my youngest son's graduation and his 21st birthday. I love my eldest son who wants me to make Chapattis for him. I love all my children too much. I love my husband the most. He means everything to me. I don't know what I would have done without him.

I want everybody to pray for me that's all.

I know my sisters and brothers love me and I love them too.

I love my father very much, dearly from my heart, and I love Daddy who I stayed with until I got married. Thank God Allah gave me two dads. Thank you.

I love my Mum so much. Nobody will ever take her place in my heart. She has a place in my heart. She did so much for me.

My friends and your aunties have done so much for me and mean so much to me. They helped me day and night. I don't know how to repay them but hopefully we can all gather when I get home. I want to thank everyone who is helping us."

I will cherish that cassette tape forever. I had the feeling Mum knew this was a chance for her to tell us what she wanted us to know. It's one of the best memories to have simply because her voice is on it. I am only sorry that it was her final message to us all. Did she know her life was at risk at this point? I would say she did.

I felt let down by the hospitals in London. It's as if the consultant who was responsible for Mum in the first week was the only angel with wings sheltering our family. He was on holiday for the second week she was there. When there was finally a slot for Mum to be operated on, we walked with her while they rolled her on the hospital bed to the lifts. Then we left so that Daddy could be briefly with her on his own before they took her to the operating room. She went in for her operation in the morning. Nobody came to talk to us to give an update.

We waited for the entire day until the surgeon finally emerged in the afternoon. He was literally about to exit the hospital to leave when Daddy recognised him and ran after him. We had been waiting for him or anyone else to give us some news the whole day. Daddy stopped him to ask what was happening with Mum. The surgeon looked at Daddy and then said that Mum had to be resuscitated three times. Then he said the septicaemia had spread to Mum's heart, which was badly infected. He said he had her heart in his hands, adding that her heart had practically fallen apart in his hands. I could have passed out at hearing that. I stopped mid-breath when I heard him say it. I can't remember taking my next breath after hearing that, only that I felt dizzy.

He was pleased his operation had been successful; that she had survived, but it wasn't clear if she would make it. He said she only had a 25% chance of surviving. We were all wondering what this meant. I wondered how we would manage back home in case she got an infection. Only positive thoughts were needed, not that thought.

The Day We Never Wanted

During the first week after she had her surgery to replace her heart valve, she was in intensive care. Soon after the operation, when she woke up, she was strong enough to say to my oldest brother, Abbid, while connected to the tubes, "Take me home." It was hard for him to see her with all these tubes attached to her, knowing he couldn't fulfil her wishes. We were all sad we couldn't honour her wish. We thought she wanted to go home to the Royal Berkshire Hospital in Reading.

She was in such terrible pain, but no more morphine was to be given to her for fear that it would reduce her chances of survival. We still believed she would somehow pull through and that she would come home, despite all that she had been through. We believed it. It felt foreign not to. Our brains had been wired to believe she was going to make it.

Mum Was Fighting To Hold On

We drew the letters of the alphabet on paper. She used her eyes when she couldn't talk to stare at the letters to simply spell out her question. "What did the Doctor say?" We explained what we had been told.

The consultant who was in charge, who we felt had done a good job taking care of her, was away for the second week. Just when we thought she was showing some signs of getting stronger, she started to decline. It turns out she wasn't improving. Eventually, it got late. One of the members of staff informed us that she was struggling.

Our family had hope, but that night we didn't go home, staying close by the hospital in London at a school friend's flat. A friend of mine from school with a big heart could see how we needed help. She had offered us her place to stay for the night, which was a beautiful thing for her to do. To see our family in distress, her offer to help us out at that difficult time meant the world to me.

Our friends knew things were not okay because they had been there throughout our Mum's journey with us. We were not contactable, since at the hospital, you couldn't use mobile phones. They were amazing to us, showing us so much love. They were great support, helping us whenever we needed it. But they knew it was a critical time for all of us. It turns out we were desperate as Mum was fighting for her life.

Darkness had overshadowed light. It was 3 February 2001. Mum had spent the last two weeks in the High Dependency Unit, specifically a place also known as the Intensive Care Unit. A one-way ticket for some.

In the morning, when we got to the hospital again, the staff informed us that Mum was in room seven. They said there was nothing more they could offer her and that it was only a matter of time. We were told at 1:30 pm on 3 February 2001, that the time had come. Mum was dying. Abbid ran to the toilet to vomit. We were all dying to see her. I vividly recall constantly being refused entry to where she had been moved to – room number seven: not everyone's lucky number.

Patients tended to be admitted to the open ward upon arrival at the hospital. They were only being moved to rooms with closed doors to give families more privacy when the outcome was bleak because their lives were ending. Mum was now in one of these rooms. We were waiting outside to be let in, thinking they were expecting us. I decided to go ahead and look through the door.

You find yourself in a trance in this sort of situation. I wasn't being rational. My rationality included assessing how she was being handled. I was comparing the care Mum had in Reading versus London, but it was irrational. In these situations it's normal to compare, so I did.

We were told she had suffered internal bleeding. The nurses asked us if we wanted to stop giving her more units of blood since it wasn't going to help her live. Nobody was pressuring us. The nurses were being patient as we took our time deciding what to do. Eventually, after lots of thought, we agreed they should stop giving it to her.

With this news, we were given time to spend with her for however long it was going to take for her to die, for her lease for life to end. Her life couldn't be saved. It was tragic. It was unbearable when I realised we were losing her. The waiting was over, but not for a kidney. This was not how we expected it to end. All our hopes for saving Mum's life were gone.

If we knew that Mum wasn't going to make it, how I wish she would have had the choice of dying at the hospital in her hometown, at the Royal Berkshire hospital in Reading, amongst the kind staff that had looked after her for ten years. They had done a brilliant job at making her comfortable. We knew she was in good hands with them. She would have been more comfortable in her last weeks, knowing she was where she wanted to be. Unfortunately, it wasn't to be.

Eventually, we were allowed to go into room seven. When I looked at Mum, she had a small tear in her eye. We stood by her bedside. She was lying very still. We all took it in turns to talk to her, like we had been doing anyway.

Mum wasn't ready to go. She was fighting to stay with us, to stay with her husband, to stay with her children, to stay living in life. I wondered how it must have felt for her to be the one dying, to be watching her family lament losing her. It must have been gut-wrenching for her to watch us all. It was an unimaginable feeling that made me tearful. It made my heart ache. Oh, how it ached. I was no longer strong or hopeful. I was crushed.

Somehow, Aneesa and I found ourselves singing one of our favourite songs to her. It was "The Sound of Silence" by Simon and Garfunkel. In contrast, she had managed to sing Happy Birthday to my younger brother, who had turned twenty-one years old only a few days earlier.

The intensive care nurses cried with us. They were compassionate people. We spent this final day with Mum until 9:37 p.m. Then it was over. We looked at the machine, where we could all see her heartbeat getting slower. Eventually, the line on the screen went flat. She had left us. She had died. She had gone. At that moment, a little part of each of us died too. Our hearts were broken into a million pieces. I cried a waterfall of tears, which became a collective sea of tears between us all. It was awful. It hurt like hell.

Gratitude Amidst Grief

I was thankful that the five of us were together during this tragic time. We remained together during these difficult times like iron filings attracted to a magnet. Abbid often quoted Mum, "You four strong children are like four straws which when put together makes you stronger. Together you are stronger." Mum was right.

It was past 1:30 a.m. in the morning by the time the last relatives had come to see her after we had informed them that she had died. I was thankful to my amazing, loving relatives. When we saw them at the hospital, we could all see the look of shock in their eyes. No one expects to see a loved one who has passed away, but here they were. Few words were spoken; instead, I could feel the heaviness in their hearts. It was surreal. I watched the looks in their eyes, the sadness as they reconciled with what had happened. They had known Mum for three decades of their lives. There she lay, clearly far too young to leave them all so soon. I longed for reality to be different, but it couldn't be changed. Ever.

By the early hours of the morning, we were shattered, with nothing left to give. We had been offered a single room for all five of us to sleep in. The five of us managed to somehow squeeze ourselves into a room that had been offered to us that night.

I knew Mum had been moved on her own to the cool freezer. I remember seeing the zip on the black bag, which poked out slightly over the white cloth that had been placed over it, when more relatives came to see her the following morning. I remember touching her skin which was cold. It made me feel sick in my stomach.

Chapter 9
The Funeral

Let's Begin at the End. 2001 Final Goodbyes

Over the next few days, some of Mum's family arrived from Canada and Kuwait. I can't imagine how it must have been for them to say goodbye to her with her being that young. She had, after all, turned fifty only two months earlier. Mum's exceptionally close group of friends, the aunties, also extended their support, their love, and their hearts to each of us children and to Daddy too. They were also amazing during the entire ordeal. They immediately stepped up to take on different responsibilities, organizing our home so we could accommodate the vast numbers of visitors. There was food, so much food for those who had come to pay their respects. They continuously checked that us girls were doing ok. They cried as we held onto them, while they told us that they had lost one of their best friends.

One friend took care of the coffin that Mum was to be placed in. She had very carefully considered the shape of it. I was impressed that she had opted for one with a rectangular shape. Not the design that you would see Dracula in. The only thing I struggled with was the smell of it, which was sandalwood. That smell hit me. It was a smell only associated with Mum's coffin. To this day, I get this block since it isn't a common smell around me, but it immediately takes me right back to seeing her lay in the coffin. I struggled with the smell of incense too, which was burned a lot during the time Mum died. It felt so intrusive, following me everywhere. It was such a strong reminder that death was around me that day. It made me want to cry, but I couldn't make it go away either. The smell lingered around me everywhere I went, which was annoying.

The day of the funeral had arrived. Visitors had come to our house to pay their respects to Mum earlier that morning, just before the prayers at the mosque. We decided to bring Mum home one last time before she was laid to rest because she hadn't been there since 7 December when she was taken to the hospital.

She was transported past the gate to the garden so that she could be carefully moved into the living room, where people could say goodbye to her quietly in their own time. It was a chance for them to have their personal moment with her. Afterwards, at the mosque, with so many people there, it was going to be hard to have a private moment to say goodbye. Then she was carefully transported into the hearse to be taken to the mosque for the service.

My cousins were brilliant, not only to Mum, but to all of us. They were kind, considerate, thoughtful, compassionate, caring, and full of love – so much love. I remember one cousin saying, "No one expected the inevitable to happen, but it did." I felt frozen with paralysis from any thoughts entering my mind as I homed in deeply to what she had said. Her words were exactly right, impacting me hard. It was like when a high-speed train passes in front of you. You feel the pull from it passing in front of you; then again as the back of the train continues past you. Your body moves slightly with it, only to be pushed back to its original position leaving you momentarily shaken.

There were hundreds of people at the mosque. The time escaped me for a minute or two. The sun struck a beam of warmth onto the ground while I stood by the hearse that was transporting Mum. My heart yearned not to be there. It was horrifying to realise that all the events were real, even the pale yellow and pink flowers against the dark black vehicle. The colourful flowers were laid across the hearse as beautifully as one could allow beauty on this sullen occasion. The sun was out, but I felt no warmth or heat. I was almost shivering with cold, even though it was warm.

The tears that had left a sticky wetness on my face were creating short-pathed tracks as they streamed down my cheeks, which usually smile. Inside, I was cold, trembling with fear. We kept being told not to cry near Mum for now was the toughest time for her since she was starting her onward journey out of this life and world. People said don't cry now because it is during this time that she will be taken on to her new journey, where her new time with God is decided.

I didn't look up. I recited prayers in my head quickly, making sure they all got to her. I had to do my bit, for as her daughter, my prayers counted very strongly, yet somehow, in the back of my head, were the words to a song I had sung with the Central Berkshire Girls' Choir called, *The Turtle Dove* by Ralph Vaughan Williams. The lyrics reminded me Mum had gone away. Worse still, she wasn't coming back. I recited the prayers, but these songs with English lyrics found their way into my head. I felt as if no wounds could be healed in me because of the gaps that had been formed by death. Then words to Bridge Over Troubled Water by Simon and Garfunkel came into my head because tears were in my eyes. Mum wasn't there to comfort me anymore. Nor was I able to comfort her. She was crying too. It felt like the tear in the duct of her eye was gathering her cries of sadness. When I thought of that tear, I saw the sea of sadness overflowing with devastation; we could all feel her sadness too.

No words could comfort me. Pain was all around. It was excruciating. It was everywhere. It split through my heart slowly like a sharp piercing. It was a bit like that burning feeling you get when you are running for a train. You find your lungs getting this burning sensation around the whole of the chest cavity. You can't get enough air into your lungs. It hurts. It really hurts. Death hurts. I felt like I had experienced it even though I wasn't the one who died. Yet it felt like a part of me had died. There was no help available at that moment to make it better because nobody could bring Mum back. She was gone. There was emotional support, yes, but nothing could stop the deep raw pain I felt. The shock, the numbness, the paralysis, the static feeling of being stuck stayed for such a long time.

I stood surrounded by the warm sun, although I dared not look up to see it beaming gloriously down onto the enormous crowd of around one hundred people. There was an even split of the mourners, consisting of a mixture of people from all different backgrounds. The journey ahead was no longer one that living people could assist with.

The feeling I had that day was gut wrenching. It was overwhelming. It was a sickening feeling. It was anything but a happy one, for my mother was being taken away to be laid to rest in Henley Road Cemetery in a neat plot alongside a pathway that led to the primary school nearby. Birds could be heard singing. Close by, children were making their typical noise in the local school playground, which I considered to be quite ironic since Mum loved kids. It was poignant that her resting place was right next to a school where she was surrounded by the sounds of children playing.

One of the biggest shocks for me was that women or girls were not permitted in our culture to go to the cemetery, even though we knew this would be the case in advance of the occasion. Watching her being driven away from the mosque to the cemetery was really upsetting. I felt I had been denied my chance to say goodbye while she was being laid to rest. Not being permitted to see her at the cemetery was something that was hard for me to deal with. Women were not permitted to go to the cemetery because of the sounds that they made while crying. Crying was considered by some to make the journey for those who had departed harder. This was because it was a tough enough time for the person who died anyway.

Cortege Of Cars

What happened next was that at around 1 p.m. Mum was driven in the hearse, followed by the funeral cortege to the Royal Berkshire Hospital in Reading. While all the cars waited outside, the hearse that she lay in was driven slowly into the main entrance. It passed the newly opened kidney dialysis unit, which had recently been moved from Dellwood Hospital to the Royal Berkshire Hospital. The atmosphere was strikingly solemn.

We wanted the staff who had cared for her over the last ten years from the hospital or newly opened dialysis unit to be able to pay their respects. They knew Mum would be driven to the entrance of the hospital building, which is where they waited until she arrived. It was a way for them and her to say goodbye.

We went back to see some of them afterwards. Oh, how they cried. They were so sad that she hadn't made it. Sad she wasn't coming back. These amazing people had spent a decade helping to prolong her life. They were her second family. She probably spent more time with them during those years than with us.

The renal staff had seen Mum almost every other day for ten years. People die all the time, which is often what happens in hospitals, but seeing the sadness in their eyes, and the look on their faces made it impossible not to cry with them. They asked us what happened, genuinely upset at the news. We explained everything to them in detail. I could feel the compassion, and the sympathetic ears while they listened to us. It felt good. It was exactly what we needed. Perhaps because Mum had been a patient of theirs for such a long time, seeing these nurses cry made it even harder for me to swallow that she had died.

We decided as a family to drive her past the kidney dialysis unit in Reading to highlight that kidney patients were living in the hope of a life-saving transplant, showing how difficult it was to find one because of a huge lack of donors. That's what we told anyone who asked. We wanted something positive to come out of Mum's death. This was a poignant way to make people think about becoming donors. Giving blood seemed to be easy but carrying a donor card was much harder. We wanted to give some positive publicity about carrying a donor card so people could see how it could help save lives. We felt sad but not bitter, wanting to do our bit even though for us, the wait was over. Had Mum received a kidney, her life would have been so different, but we couldn't change that now.

While the men were laying Mum to rest, we made our way home. The house was full of women who were there to pray for her. This was a strong community of women who, along with their relatives, stepped in to help. They prepared the house by covering up all the photos of people's faces. Apparently, that's what you do when someone has died. There was a huge bucket with thousands of beans to count blessings for Mum. They organised everything in the house so that people could take part in these prayers or pass by to pay their respects. We invited anyone into the house who came by, since after all, our lives had been spent around relatives and friends from a mix of backgrounds. They had come from different parts of the world, including Kuwait, Canada, Pakistan, India, Saudi Arabia, Yemen, and the UK which had included our lovely neighbours from Wales.

The community had gathered at our house for one reason: to pay their respects to Mum. The aunties sat on the floor talking to us, telling us how kind Mum was to them. I felt like I had sweated through my salwar kameez, my face sticky from all the tears, which left me with puffy cheeks. I must have cried a thousand tears that day. I didn't think I could cry any more, but the tears didn't stop falling. The women who knew Mum from her community told us how "Sabiha wasn't suffering anymore." Sabiha is what the women called her, which was her name from Kuwait. Everyone else called her Annsa.

They told us their own stories of how they too lost their mothers. It made me realise that some of them were in their early twenties, like we were. A new bond had been created between us since we could relate to each other. It felt strange having to be the centre of attention in the room. Being Annsa's daughters meant all the women came to talk to us twins, which felt comforting.

I was humbled that so many people came to the house, which meant hundreds of shoes were at the front door. Shoes from different cultures were piled up at the entrance, having come from different parts of the world. When our brothers got back, we immediately went upstairs with them, desperate to know what happened at the cemetery. Abbid said he never imagined he would have to bury his mother so soon. He explained how Mum was lowered into the ground and how they all buried her. I could see the pain in his eyes from every part he described to us.

When people came to our house, including on the day of the funeral, we tried to get the women to listen to us. We wanted to get that conversation going to help them understand that more people from ethnic minority communities needed to be organ donors. It was a sensitive situation, which made it difficult. The women were from different parts of the world and were all sitting in the same room because of Mum. They were there to pay their respects. Although we had a captive audience, trying to hold a conversation about organ donation wasn't easy. It wasn't something they were open to hearing us talk about, especially not at a funeral. We know because we tried. It went down like a lead balloon, leaving me feeling deflated. Perhaps they thought it was disrespectful to Mum since she was literally being laid to rest. I could feel their uneasiness at being asked about it by us. We had nothing to lose by trying to talk but we remained respectful to them all. It was hard to be angry with your elders when perhaps it was us that should have tried to talk about the topic earlier. Whether or not any of them felt responsible for their inaction is not something I have pondered on. One does what one feels guided or compelled to do, and I am not going to judge anyone for not taking any action. I just wish I had said something to the community all those years earlier. Now it was too late.

I accept that for some people in the room, they were solely there to pray for Mum. It wasn't the right time or the right place to bring it up. But when is? Well, us twins must have had it in us to say something because we couldn't sit there silently. There was no big announcement. We were just trying to break the taboo by making them aware of how hard it was to get a kidney because Mum was Asian.

Apart from one family who said they would register on the National Organ Donor Register, some women spoke back saying things like our organs should be buried with us when we die. I blurted out with a very slightly raised voice, "Then how would Mum ever get a kidney if no Asian donates? She needed an Asian donor." Didn't they understand what I said? I think they didn't. Or perhaps they didn't want to.

There was no response, just the sound of each prayer being spoken out loud, followed by a bean being placed into the huge bucket. It was incredibly frustrating. How were we supposed to get them to have a conversation about saving lives? Here we were sitting on the floor, grieving as real-life examples of daughters who had lost their mother, but no one was listening. They could hear us but were not listening. It created a tense atmosphere for a short time because they wanted to be compassionate to us, but they were clear in their opinion on the topic. This wasn't going to be discussed right now. I felt deflated, quietly joining in with the prayers for the rest of the day.

Later on, us twins went to see exactly where Mum had been laid to rest. I felt like she was constantly around me. It didn't feel to me like she was at the cemetery. I felt like her soul was free, like she was in the sky. Whenever the sun shone out, I would say, Sun's out, Mum's out. That made it a little easier since nature is around us. It is everywhere. I was lucky enough to have her in my dreams. She looked healthy every time. We hugged each other, talking lots. I even said to her, "I guess you have to go back to heaven now," in my dream. I would wake up telling my family that she was in my dream. They would say how lucky I was. It was the best feeling ever to wake up knowing there was a small connection that felt real.

The next few weeks were spent gathering her salwar kameezes that we didn't want to keep. Soon enough, over one hundred huge bags of her clothes had been filled to pass on to Charity. We took her remaining medication to the pharmacy to dispose of. The staff remembered her, expressing their condolences.

We listened to music that made us cry, laugh, and sing together to make it less painful. We kept Mum's favourite handbag that she took to dialysis. Her wedding ring was rotated between us children, her dinner sets from her time at school in Kuwait that she won as prizes were divided amongst us. Each time she did well, she was presented with a dinner set, a tea set, or drinking glasses.

Now, when we eat certain meals on an occasion that means something to me, I set the table, bringing out the dinner set every time to celebrate Mum. I converted the cassette tape of her speaking into an MP3, listening to her voice repetitively. I spent time going to my aunties' houses to be around people who talked about her. They talked, telling stories of their time with her, which brought me so much happiness.

They took care of me while I was completely at a loss for what to do with myself now that Mum wasn't there anymore. They fed me, letting me cry into their arms. They showered me with love to make up for the massive hole that had been left in my heart. There was a funny food moment with the family amid the sadness when we sat down to eat dinner together without Mum for the first time. Someone asked if anyone wanted the doner kebab in the fridge that was still there. One of us replied, "Donor? It's a bit late for that now, isn't it?"

We found ourselves rolling our eyes, not knowing whether to laugh or cry, but somehow it broke the tension we had been living with for such a long time. I had now entered a new part of life without Mum in it. Who was going to support Daddy, given the bond they had? How were we going to manage life when we were older without having Mum to talk to? Daddy was of course there too, but since he worked all the time at the shop, it was Mum that I used to telephone at university to get advice from about how to mix the spices perfectly for the food I was cooking. Who was going to show the same level of interest when there was some news going on in my life? Suddenly there was a whole bunch of "how's" or "what ifs", all because of this almighty gap that appeared because Mum wasn't there to turn to anymore.

Campaigning After Mum Died

Following Mum's death, we jumped into gear to try to raise awareness about organ donation. The local TV station, Meridien TV, came over to interview us for their 5 p.m. program. The presenters did a really great job at showing sensitivity towards us while listening to our story about how our mother of four had lost her fight for life.

We even took out a pile of organ donor cards that we had picked up at the local pharmacy so that we could give them to anyone who wanted one. I was quite dismayed at how many times people politely said they didn't want one. Aneesa even formed a choir at university, which she called the Kidney Choir, to raise money from the concerts for the dialysis unit in Reading.

Journalists from the Reading Evening Post[13] newspaper came to our house the following week to interview us about Mum. They wrote a double-page spread highlighting that there were declining numbers of donors in the Asian community.

I had written letters to The Times newspaper in 2001[14] and to the London Metro newspaper in 2002, which got published. I, like my family, slowly started to do my part, in raising awareness about the need for organ donation. The best thing about these articles is knowing that the issue I was writing about for twenty years did see a change in the law regarding the soft opt-out, since this will make some difference.

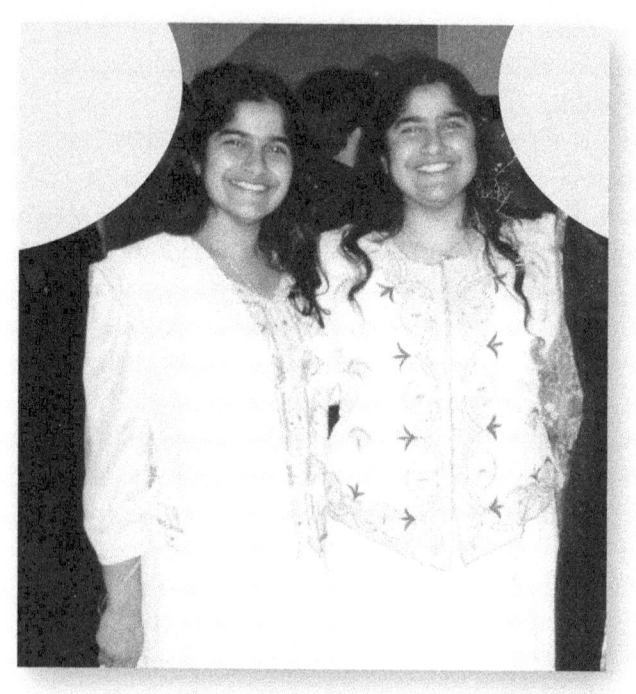

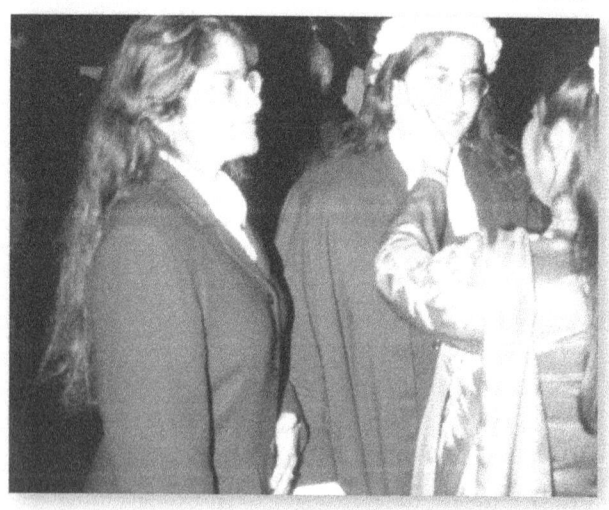

Chapter 10
Life Now

Without Mum

I was travelling around Northern Ireland and the Republic of Ireland in 2019 when I found myself in Dublin at a Desi Indian restaurant. I opted for my favourite: mincemeat and peas. I got quietly excited because I had almost never seen that on a restaurant menu. I decided to try it. I ordered it with two chapattis right away, waiting curiously. I wondered how it might taste since it had been decades since I had eaten this dish – a dish Mum knew was a favourite of mine and loved to cook for me. The ingredients were fresh, the peas were not from a tin. When I started to eat it, my eyes suddenly filled with tears. I had the biggest cry ever. It lasted for a ridiculously, embarrassingly long time. It was the first time something had triggered a memory of Mum's food that left me feeling hugely emotional since it tasted so good.

I can, of course, cook some of the dishes I learned to cook from Mum, like her Pakistani chicken, but other dishes just don't taste the same. Once I had finished crying, I composed myself and asked the waitress to thank the chef. She thought I was crying because it was too spicy. It wasn't. It was delicious, going straight to my heart. All the feelings of my mother's love came flowing right back into my heart. It felt full of Mum's warmth again, for that short time. It was such a beautiful feeling. Yes, it was emotional, but it was like breathing air that she had filled with hugs, love, and warmth. I went back the next day, ordering exactly the same dish again. It still tasted so good. When they asked me if I wanted it a little extra spicy, I had to say no because the way it tasted was how Mum cooked it for us kids. My heart was happy.

Final Thoughts

I hope that by reading about this chapter of my life, you take some time to think about my message. I ask you to please pause for more than a moment while you are distracted by the material needs of this beautiful but cruel world. Consider my message: What would it be like if this were to happen to you or to someone close to you?

While writing this memoir, it has felt at times like I am watching a movie, fearing getting to the end whilst knowing what is going to happen. This hasn't stopped me from trying to make it my business to help save lives by telling my story. It makes my time here on this earth worthwhile.

To quote Shakespeare's Macbeth, "What is done is done and cannot be undone." Although this is true, there is little sense in holding onto the tragedy alone. To hold onto such sadness for too long makes the simple task of breathing enormously difficult. It feels like you are suffocating yourself. I did that for a while until I gave myself permission to be happy again.

Mum often said she wanted her children to be happy. As I closed my eyes, it was easy to imagine, at least for a moment, as I lost myself in my thoughts. Imagination can be a wonderful thing when it paints happiness in your mind. It feels even better when you transfer that feeling into life. So I decided it's okay to be happy so that I could start to live my best life. I didn't want to feel lost anymore. I love to use this phrase that I came across: "Don't Dream Your Life. Live Your Dream." I truly believe that. If it is possible, despite experiencing loss, then what's stopping you?

I hope with all that I have written, you can see how saving lives in the form of a gift is not only for the person who received the gift of life but for the family too. I, for one, will continue to raise awareness about organ donation, offering support to anyone who wants to talk about it. It is only through all of these interactions that the message gets louder. Help others to live after your death. Family matters. Pass it on.

Intellectual Debate

Mum only survived for a further ten years because of dialysis, which was her lease for life. Without it, she would have died much earlier. My simple message to you reading this is this: Carry the donor card that is offered where you live as a symbol of your decision to help others. If you're in the UK, register your decision on the Organ Donation Register and talk to your family about your decision. The people who receive your organs will be happy. I promise.

I know from listening to stories that life can be hard even after a transplant, but wouldn't it have been great to have that chance? Life for those families waiting for a transplant would be so different. Had Mum gotten a kidney, I would have loved to talk to her, especially during my later adult life, about what decisions to make, where to live, what career path to take, where to go on holiday, and how to carry on celebrating life with her. She would have loved to meet her grandchildren. She would have flown across the world to do it.

Today, many communities, including my own, are still not speaking up enough about organ donation. This is detrimental to the survival of so many ethnic communities out there. Be different. Take a stand, speak up. Tell your stories. We need to tell our stories. They need to be heard.

Yes, there is some variation in the opinions of religious scholars on donation. I wish to highlight the scholars speaking at webinars from the British Islamic Medical Association[15] whose guidance makes clear that it is acceptable to donate if this helps to save a life. Surely donating can also be seen considered to be doing good? See it as a good deed if you will or see it as a form of charity, something that is helping someone. It can even be considered permissible because saving a life is a principle necessity.

The irony, at least for my community, is that our parents want their children to be doctors. Interestingly, Asian parents seem to be fine with their children having the title of doctor, which usually means saving lives. Isn't the work that they are doing even more important than the title? Now there are many more Asian doctors promoting organ donation because they know there is a lack of donation in their own communities. They sit with patients in their suffering or at the end stages of their lives. They can see with their own eyes how certain communities of people are dying faster because they have dug their own hole by refusing consent for their deceased loved ones to be organ donors. My hope is that people in different ethnic communities will listen to people from their own backgrounds when they are confronted with the question of donation.

My impression is that people find it easier to distance themselves from donation when they don't know who the patient is. They are more likely to say they want to help because someone they know needs a life-saving transplant. These people argue that they would be a living donor to a family member but not to anyone else. They would still rather be buried along with their organs when they die than to have donated at death. To that, I say, think bigger than yourself. This affects not only you, but your family and the generations that will follow who will face the same barriers.

Humanity doesn't naturally help itself here, but it so easily could. When you see domestic pets at home suffer, they can be treated for a short while. Sometimes, to prevent their suffering, they get put down. For some people, losing a pet is almost as heartbreaking as losing a human loved one. I can relate to that regarding my cats. They broke my heart when they died. Yet humans are the only species on this planet that have the ability to help each other survive for longer. We have made massive strides in medical advances to improve our quality of life or to save it. But if the speed of progress continues at this snail's pace, then not only will we be too slow to help the older generation, but ours and the ones that follow us will face the impact too.

Mistrust in the medical profession hasn't helped the cause either. I understand that in some communities, people from certain backgrounds were wrongly taken advantage of for medical advancement. The medical sector has a history of mistreating Black Americans — from horrific experiments on enslaved people to forced sterilisations of Black women, not to mention the Tuskegee syphilis study that withheld treatment from hundreds of Black men in the US for decades to let doctors track the course of the disease. It was 100% wrong. I saw how, during the COVID pandemic that began in 2020, certain communities had a similar mistrust. I understood this too. However, that doesn't detract from the current problems of today regarding the lack of people donating where they would be helping to save a life either while living or after they died.

Further mistrust came from hospital scandals. The Alder Hey Hospital organs scandal was a case in the UK where, without authorization organs had been removed, kept in jars, or disposed of. This included body parts from around 850 infants. This happened in 1996 when Mum had already been waiting for a kidney for around five years. It's hard to ask people to be sympathetic to your cause when you read about these awful cases in the media.

Eurotransplant is an ethical international organ-exchange organisation that covers countries in Europe, including Austria, Belgium, Croatia, Germany, Hungary, Luxemburg, the Netherlands, and Slovenia. There have been many partners involved in the organ exchange process, such as transplant hospitals, tissue-typing laboratories, hospitals where organ donations take place, and national competent authorities. The

Eurotransplant region has a population of approximately 135 million people.

In 2013, the organisation noticed from their records that wrongful activity was taking place by the medical profession, which led to an investigation. Several transplant centres across Germany had allegedly manipulated donor waiting lists[16], which were then under criminal investigation. Doctors had falsified the level of illness of a patient. It gave patients access to donor organs not only quicker but ahead of other patients in Europe who were part of an organ-exchange system through Eurotransplant.

Those cases resulted in accusations of corruption in the system, which led to massive mistrust by the public. It's exactly this German scandal that I heard about when I asked people in Germany who were from the same ethnic background as mine about their view on organ donation. The general opinion was that the organ donation scandals were something that could easily have been avoided. Some people could only ever contemplate donation if they were a living donor for their family member. At least that way, the organ would go to who they actually wanted it to go to, rather than to someone who needed it but paid to get pushed up the list. To these people, it really mattered who their organs went to. With other organs, unlike the kidney, you don't need to check for tissue typing therefore making it easier for this sort of wrongful activity to happen.

I explained how my family was a perfect example because we tried to be living donors, but it didn't work because for kidney transplants, there must be a match from the blood group and tissue typing. That's why we had to wait so long for a donor from the same background to donate, which never happened. The conversation ended abruptly.

The damage that these scandals have done, even though it was a few isolated incidents, has been huge. The result has been that this small handful of cases led to a decrease of between 20% to 40% in the number of Germans willing to donate organs directly after the scandals.

People are still concerned that if they are asked to donate their deceased loved ones' organs, the doctors might speed up their death. One must have trust in the system. Otherwise, you may as well not use it when you need it. All I can say is that if you have told your family about your wishes to donate and registered your intent on the register, then hopefully they would honour your wishes.

That's why it is important for stories like mine to be told. Although these stigmas are valid, there are still plenty of normal, honest patients who simply want an improvement in their quality of life.

One must look at the other perspective that people see. Altruism. Why is it that there are people in this world who have this overwhelming urge to help donate to people they don't even know while they are still alive? They don't even think that much about it. That blows my mind away. These people are known as altruistic people. They are heroes. They don't see it like that, though. I personally don't know anyone in my community who is quite that altruistic. I am hopeful that they are out there. To donate in principle anonymously is easier than letting your loved ones know what you are doing. Since you are donating anonymously, you don't even know where your organs are going. That is incredibly humble.

Let's help each other to live! How else will this problem ever be overcome? We must talk to each other without being afraid of upsetting the people we are talking to. I have hope that those of you who opted out of your automatic entry to the Organ Donation Register will now consider opting back in. Your selflessness, not selfishness, will save lives. Your decision to give life to others so they can live life will keep families together for longer. Remember, family matters! Don't forget!

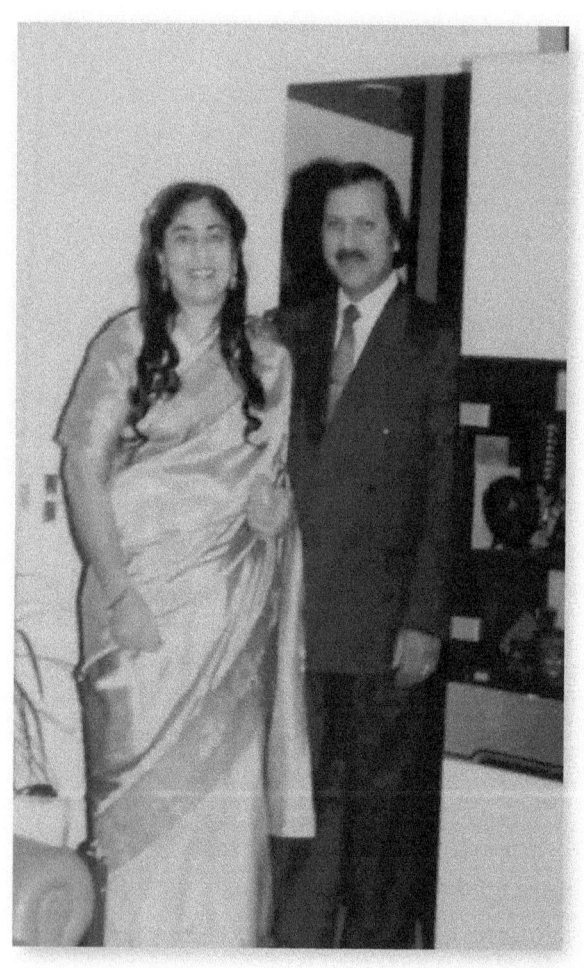

Acknowledgments

To my father Ajaz Chaudhry for letting me into your life without Mum and for letting you into mine with your heart. You surprised me with your openness, and I learn from you every day.

To my relatives and friends of Mum who provided love and support all the way through.

To my writer's coach Ali Bagley: I literally may never have picked up this memoir and completed it had I not met you. I am grateful.

To Angee Khan, Alia Tayer and Hoda Malone for supporting me with the editing, transitions, and flows.

Thanks to Emily, Abbid, Smruti, Aneesa, Petra and Katie for your feedback.

Heartfelt gratitude to transplant surgeon Dale Gardiner from the NHS, for providing me with facts and enabling me to obtain data representing South Asian, Arab, Black, and Chinese country data.

To Simonne Weeks from University of Brighton Donor Research Team for your support.

Thanks to sponsors Hilary Rose and Anita Myers.

Thanks to Fr. Biju Peter, Mini Karuppan and Bhindu Xavier for contributions on donation success stories.

Finally, I want to express my gratitude to my friends and family for all your support and encouragement over the past 23 years. I will be forever grateful.

A. S. Chaudhry.
Berlin, Germany December 2024

Facts and Information on Organ Donation

My story only covers people from the smaller minority groups in the UK. The law is different in each country so I would encourage anyone reading, to investigate how to donate where you live.

You can register your decision in the UK here:
https://www.organdonation.nhs.uk/ register-your-decision/

You can register your decision in Germany here:
https://www.ueber-leben.de/organspendeausweis/#kostenlos-bestellen

Organ donation and your beliefs:

The NHS in the UK is committed to working with faith leaders and representatives of the various beliefs systems in the UK.

https://www.organdonation.nhs.uk/helping-you-to-decide/your-faith-and-beliefs/

Does organ donation affect burial?

After donation, the body is returned to the family of the deceased in the same way as any death in a hospital where donation has not taken place. The family is then free to make whatever arrangements they feel appropriate. Donation does not delay this happening. This means a family can make decisions about the burial without worrying about a delay due to respecting the deceased's wishes to donate. I find this information reassuring and see it as a win-win since the wishes of the deceased are respected, and at the same time the family can plan for burial in accordance with their faith and beliefs.

Figure 1: UK potential organ donor population, by ethnic minority groups, 1.4.2022-31.3.2023.

Reprint of Figure 1.1 page 11 of the publicly available *"NHS Blood and Transplant Annual Report on Ethnicity Differencesin Organ Donation and Transplantation"*

UK Population	~67,300,000
UK Deaths	~660,000
Deaths in hospitals	~290,000
All potential donors	6763
Potential ethnic minority donors	750
Referred potential ethnic minority donors	711
Ethnic minority donation requests	359
Consented ethnic minority donors	125
Actual ethnic minority donors	246*
Ethnic minority transplant patients	1106*
Ethnic minority transplants	1128*
Ethnic minority waiting list	2237

*Please note that 138 living donors have been included in this figure

Figure 2: Percentage that are ethnic minority relative to the population, 1.4.2022-31.3.2023.

The figure shows an overrepresentation of people from ethnic minority backgrounds relative to the population of England and Wales for Organ Donor Register (ODR) opt-outs, those on the waiting list, deceased donor transplants and living donor transplants. Ethnic minority groups are under-represented in deceased donors as well as eligible deceased donors, living donors and those registering on the opt-in ODR.

Reprint of Figure 1.3, page 15 of the publicly available *"NHS Blood and Transplant Annual Report on Ethnicity Differences in Organ Donation and Transplantation"*

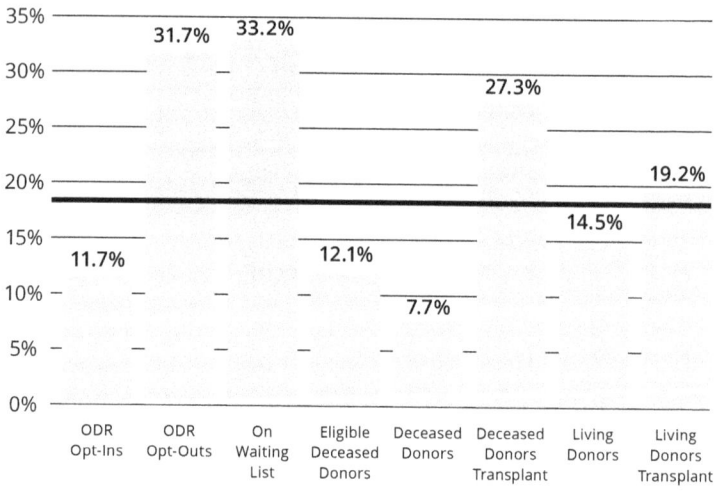

Figure 3: International Transplant Rates.

Figures created from data on pages 58 to 61 in the publicly available Council of Europe Newsletter Transplant International figures on donation and transplantation 2022 EDQM Volume 28

https://www.transplant-observatory.org/wp-content/uploads/2023/10/NEWSLETTER-2023-baja.pdf

Total number of patients transplanted
(kidney, liver, heart, heart-lung, pancreas, small bowel)
(people per million population 2023)

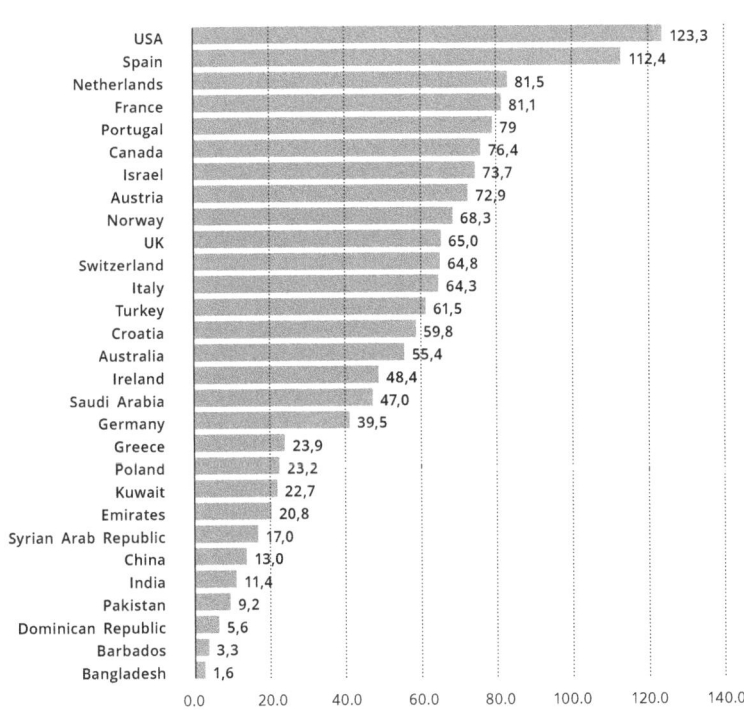

Figure 4: Kidney donations rates from deceased donors internationally.

Figures created from data on pages 58 to 61 in the publicly available Council of Europe Newsletter Transplant International figures on donation and transplantation 2022 EDQM Volume 28

https://www.transplant-observatory.org/wp-content/uploads/2023/10/NEWSLETTER-2023-baja.pdf

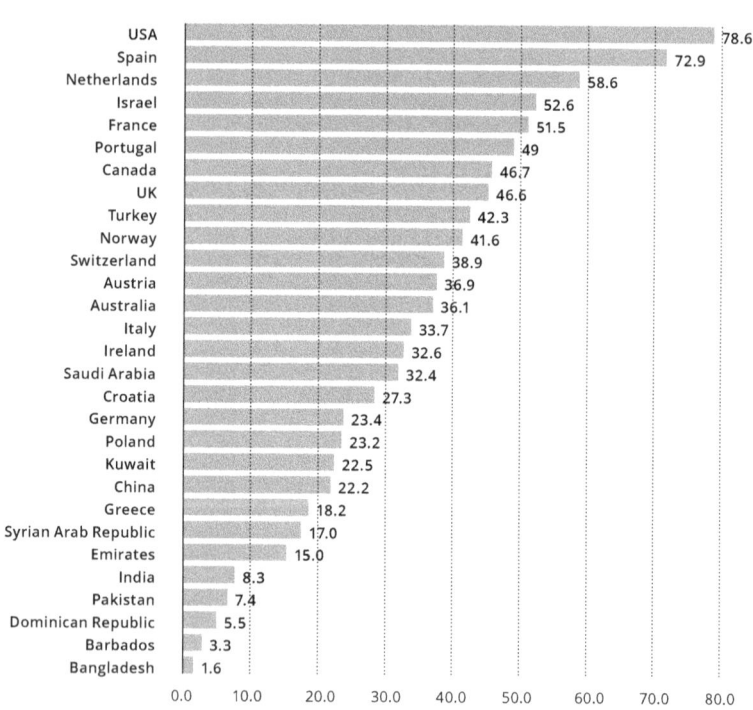

Kidney donations rates from deceased donors internationally (people per million population 2023)

USA	78.6
Spain	72.9
Netherlands	58.6
Israel	52.6
France	51.5
Portugal	49
Canada	46.7
UK	46.6
Turkey	42.3
Norway	41.6
Switzerland	38.9
Austria	36.9
Australia	36.1
Italy	33.7
Ireland	32.6
Saudi Arabia	32.4
Croatia	27.3
Germany	23.4
Poland	23.2
Kuwait	22.5
China	22.2
Greece	18.2
Syrian Arab Republic	17.0
Emirates	15.0
India	8.3
Pakistan	7.4
Dominican Republic	5.5
Barbados	3.3
Bangladesh	1.6

Table 1: Reasons for family's refusal to give consent/authorise to organ donation by ethnicity, 1.4.2018-31.3.2023.

Reprint of Table 3.3 of the "NHS Blood and Transplant Annual Report on Ethnicity Differences in Organ Donation and Transplantation"

Consent/authorisation refusal reason	Potential Donor Ethnicity									
	White		Asian		Black		Mixed		Other	
	N	%	N	%	N	%	N	%	N	%
Patient had previously expressed a wish not to donate	1054	28.2	115	19.7	69	23.2	2	5.4	14	15.9
Family were not sure whether the patient would have agreed to donation	530	14.2	55	9.4	39	13.1	3	8.1	13	14.8
Family felt the length of time for the donation process was too long	505	13.5	13	2.2	8	2.7	2	5.4	5	5.7
Family did not want surgery to the body	332	8.9	52	8.9	19	6.4	4	10.8	12	13.6
Family felt patient had suffered enough	330	8.8	21	3.6	14	4.7	4	10.8	2	2.3
Other	289	7.7	37	6.3	15	5.0	5	13.5	8	9.1
Family divided over the decision	155	4.1	15	2.6	9	3.0	4	10.8	1	1.1
Strong refusal - probing not appropriate	123	3.3	19	3.3	8	2.7	2	5.4	5	5.7
Family felt that the body should be buried whole*	109	2.9	24	4.1	18	6.0	2	5.4	5	5.7
Family did not believe in donation	97	2.6	24	4.1	12	4.0	2	5.4	2	2.3
Patient had registered a decision to Opt Out	65	1.7	25	4.3	15	5.0	1	2.7	2	2.3
Family wanted to stay with the patient after death	52	1.4	1	0.3	1	2.7				
Family felt it was against their religious/cultural beliefs	45	1.2	172	29.5	60	20.1	4	10.8	19	21.6
Family concerned that organs may not be transplantable	31	0.8	2	0.3						
Family concerned other people may disapprove/be offended	7	0.2	4	0.7	5	1.7	1	2.7		
Family had difficulty understanding/accepting neurological testing	6	0.2	2	0.3	3	1.0				
Family concerned donation may delay the funeral	4	0.1	4	0.7						
Family concerned about organ allocation	3	0.1	2	0.7						
Family believe patient's treatment may have been limited to facilitate organ donation	2	0.1	1	0.3						
Total	3739	100.0	584	100.0	298	100.0	37	100.0	88	100.0

* (unrelated to religious/cultural reasons)

Footnote References

1) Baxter comparison of dialysis types.
https://bit.ly/3AKj4NG

2) Dialysis: an introduction to dialysis.
https://bit.ly/3SX2Bw3

Both methods have their advantages. In both types, the principle is the same: a cleaning fluid (called dialysate) is used to take the impurities, salt, and water away from the blood. The impurities pass from the blood into the cleaning fluid. There has to be a barrier between the blood and the cleaning fluid for this to happen. In haemodialysis, the barrier is the filter in the dialysis machine that the blood passes through and in peritoneal dialysis, the barrier is the layer of cells that lines the abdomen and covers the intestines (the peritoneum).

3) The Organ Donation (Deemed Consent) Act 2019 known as Max and Keira's Law in honour of a nine-year-old boy who received a heart transplant and the nine -year-old girl who donated it.

4) NHS Blood and Transplant Annual Report on Ethnicity Differences in Organ Donation and Transplantation, page 5.
https://bit.ly/4g4Eq8H

5) How the opt out system works. **https://bit.ly/4dEN8ZV**

6) & 7) The Council of Europe Transplant Newsletter International figures on donation and transplantation 2022.
https://bit.ly/4g0uiOv

8) The Gunpowder plot of 1605 was when Guy Fawkes and Catholic conspirators attempted to blow up Parliament and assassinate James I of England. To celebrate his survival, King James ordered the people of England to have a bonfire on

the night of 5 November. All over Britain, there are firework displays and bonfires with models of Guy Fawkes that are burned on the fire.

9) Southall was often called Little Punjab or Little India in West London. It has been a highly populated South Asian hub since the 1950's.

10) Normal veins are not strong enough for dialysis because blood is pumped through the dialysis machine at high speeds. A 'stronger' blood vessel needs to be created. A fistula is a connection that is made by connecting a vein to an artery either in the wrist area or upper arm. This creates a large, robust blood vessel that can be needled regularly for use during haemodialysis

11) German Reference Centre for Ethics in the Life Sciences (2022): In Focus: Organ Transplantation.
https://bit.ly/471EhPc
The United Nations (UN) and the World Health Organization (WHO), reject any commercialization of organ donation, citing human rights – even though the shortage of organs is increasingly leading to illegal trafficking.

12) A set of chambers is the name for barristers who join together to share the costs of practicing law.

13) READING EVENING POST, Thursday, February 8, 2001. *"Waiting for the Transplant that never happened"* See Notes and references.

14) Letters to The Times, Friday March 2, 2001, Organ donors and the MAIL METRO August 12, 2002. There should be increased advertising from the government to enourage transplants. More donors needed. See Notes and References.

15) Let's Talk About Organ Donation Webinar. Islamic perspective on organ donation, Sheikh Dr Mansur Ali (Arabic

and Islamic studies lecturer at Cardiff University, special interest in Islamic ruling and ethics of organ donation. **https://bit.ly/4fZPdkG**

16) Article in The Guardian newspaper: **https://bit.ly/46ZOdsF**

Campaigning & Media
Letters to Newspapers

READING EVENING POST, Thursday, February 8, 2001

"Waiting for the Transplant that never happened"

"Annsa Sabiha Chaudhry probably would have lived if she'd had a kidney transplant. But sadly, the time ran out for the mother of four as she waited for a donor. At the time there had just been an organ scandal at another hospital so it meant there were growing concerns that donors may become increasingly scarce due to the scandal."

THE TIMES NEWSPAPER, Friday March 2, 2001 –

Letter to the Editor. Organ donors. From Ms. Aisha Chaudhry:

"Sir, I saw your e-poll. Do you carry a donor card? (Times Online, February 27, 2001). My mother, Annsa Chaudhry, passed away three weeks ago after waiting for a kidney transplant for 10 years. She was an Asian woman and mother of four.

There is a need for more people to carry donor cards, and especially those in ethnic communities. My mother's life was prolonged for a further 10 years through dialysis and we are grateful for that, but why do people find it so easy to give blood and yet find it so difficult to carry a donor card?

There should be more government advertising, and the introduction of an opt-out system stating that unless otherwise requested your organs will be donated.

It may be too late for my mother, but there is still hope for other people out there. Life is a gift. It shouldn't be taken for granted."

MAIL METRO NEWSPAPER, August 12, 2002

There should be increased advertising from the government to encourage transplants. More donors needed.

"In response to your article about the lack of organ donors (Metro, Tuesday), this issue could be dealt with positively if there were more government advertising encouraging people to carry a donor card and to register on the National Organ Donor Register. That way, for those who want to help someone to live after they die, their organs can be used for transplantation and not remain with them when the time ends. Another point would be to implement an opt out system like other countries in Europe. This means that unless you state otherwise, your organs will be used for transplantation, or get your workplace to make donor cards available. Trying to raise awareness among the community about the severe lack of organ donors will be a key goal while I am alive. My mother waited for a kidney transplant for 10 years before her fight for life ended last year. It may be too late to help her, but it's not too late to help someone else."

Donor and Recipient Success Story

Fr. Biju Peter CMI

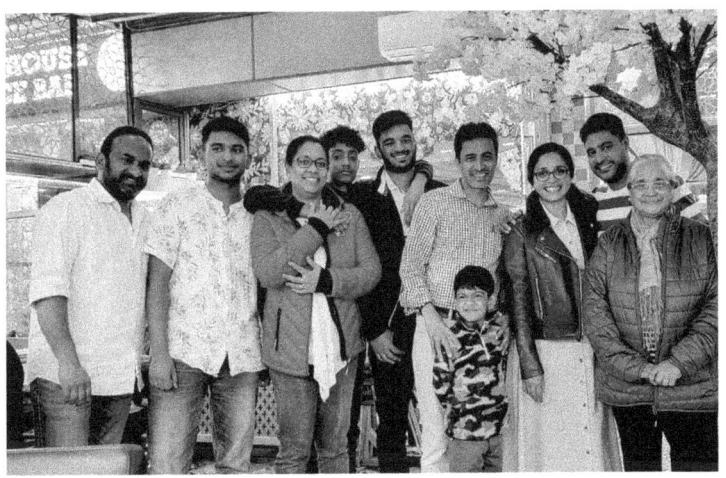

My name is Fr. Biju Peter, and I truly recognise the value and significance of organ donation. I was a recipient of a kidney transplant in May 2012, however, I consider myself particularly fortunate as my donor was my younger brother. Though my family had suspected that there was a possibility of hereditary kidney disease, it was only at the age of 27 that I was diagnosed with Polycystic Kidney Disease (PKD). My doctor recommended that rather than undergoing a dialysis procedure, a kidney transplant would be more effective, given the severity of my health issues by that point. At this time, I had moved from my native India to the United States for pastoral ministerial duties at the Blessed Sacrament Church, in New Rochelle, New York. Hence, hearing this news at such a young age alone was devastating. However, once my family heard of the update, their generosity and kindness overwhelmed me. My mother, sister and brother all live in the United Kingdom, yet they almost immediately set about being by my side during this troubling time. Although my mother was unable to come to the US, my sister and my brother joined me and we considered either of them to be prospective donors as the chance of a match would be likely. Ultimately, given my younger brother's age, we decided to go ahead with the transplant and that he would be the donor. I will never forget his sacrifice.

Following the transplant, my recuperation lasted two months over which time my siblings and I were able to also recuperate our love for each other. Since our respective childhoods, we have unfortunately all spent time apart due to our studies and work responsibilities. However, during this time, my sister, brother, and I lived together in a little house away from the city. My sister's presence was a blessing. She is an excellent cook, and so we enjoyed eating fresh Indian food. She ensured that my brother and I took the medications at the proper times, and it was she who accompanied us on our daily walks. We played cards, told jokes, shared funny stories, and reminisced about our childhood. Their company helped alleviate my isolation, and I definitely accelerated my recovery. It had been many years since my sister, brother, and I lived together as a family. This was a great consolation for me and them. I wonder if it was God's plan to gather us together to rebuild and strengthen our sibling relationships. Now when I reminisce, I thank God for giving us this blessed opportunity to become closer. Therefore, I cannot understate the importance of organ donation. It means that patients in dire need are given a new lease on life, and at least in my case, I cannot be more grateful.

Donor and Recipient Success Story

Mini Karuppan

What can I say and where do I start? My life was going by as normally as possible. Just the usual juggling between personal and professional commitments. I am a nurse and used to work in critical care. One day, whilst at work I felt generally unwell, dizzy and had the feeling that something wasn't right. My colleagues helped me, and when I checked my blood pressure it was extremely high.

A routine appointment with my doctor along with my blood results revealed that I was experiencing kidney failure. This came as a huge shock to me, as there was no family history of kidney disease. I went through an array of emotions. The feeling of frustration, anger, sadness and the constant question of WHY ME? This was a constant and it took me a while to deal with this and come to terms with my diagnosis as there was a lot to take in and prepare oneself for any eventuality. My family and friends stood by me and were a constant pillar of strength and positivity.

The next few months were spent in a daze attending hospital appointments meeting various medical teams, especially the renal team. During this phase of my life, there appeared to be numerous blood investigations, scans, X-rays, biopsies and having a fistula (in view of undergoing haemodialysis). There appeared to be rapid decline in my kidney function and in general body function. The smallest of tasks felt like a huge burden, especially with shortness of breath, extreme fatigue and a host of other signs and symptoms.

The decline in kidney function had triggered me onto

joining the organ donor list. The team had updated me that it was a 5 to 7 year wait for a transplant within the Asian community. This was most disheartening when compared to Caucasian groups who didn't have to wait this long. In the meantime, dialysis was the way forward. The journey of living life on the dialysis machine and the impact it would have on my life and that of my family was a huge burden. My husband and son were with me each and every step of the way. The positive mindset and encouragement to live life and make the best of what I could at that time helped. It propelled me into not giving up and keeping myself focused on doing things one day at a time.

Time flew by and 2 years passed by already when we are all set up to commence dialysis in the hospital. We were just waiting for a date and time schedule. I received a call assuming I was going in for dialysis. I froze when I heard that it was for a potential kidney transplant.

It has now been 6 years since I had my transplant, and I have carried on with living my life to the best of my ability.

I believe I was lucky, and it was God's plan to bond me with my donor. My faith has brought me this far and not a day goes by where I don't think about them, pray and thank them. I am forever grateful and indebted to my donor for their wonderful gift of life. I respect and carry them along with me going forward in life. I consider this a blessing and always have a warm and wonderful feeling whenever I think of them.

I accept life with all its complexities and continue to carry on living a life with eagerness and excitement. I stand as a testament of what a transplant can do in transforming a person's life. I champion organ donation and participate in campaigns to promote among Asian communities. Organ donation can change lives. It has definitely changed mine!

Donor and Recipient Success Story

Ms. Bindhu Xavier, Manchester, UK

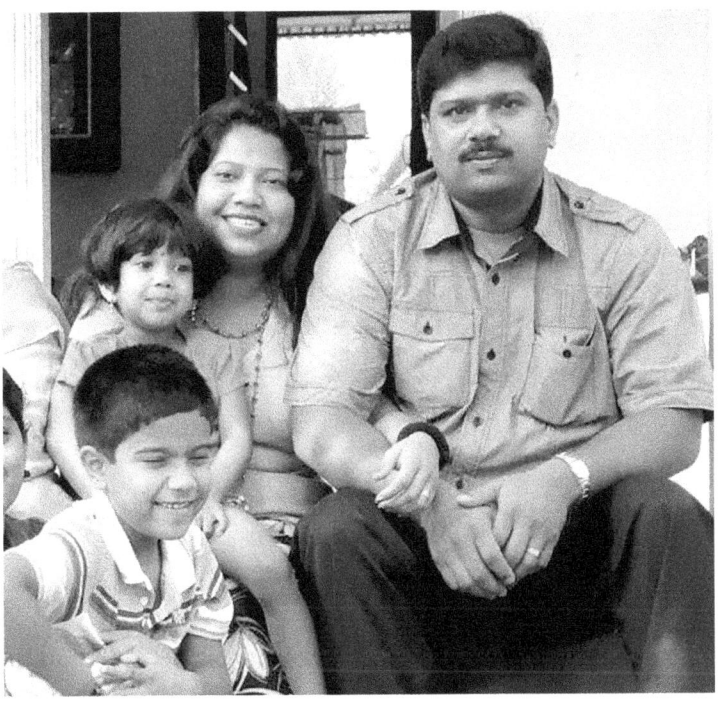

Dedicated to a beautiful soul – Brion Xavier, who is still in our midst in spirit, and my children Austin & Ashlene who give me a reason to go on every day.

My name is Bindhu & I live in Manchester with my 2 children. My background is about 18 years of Critical Care (ICU) Nursing and Research Nursing for the last 6-7 years. I was introduced to organ donation and the need for it during my ICU days. I remember one ICU shift, where unfortunately, a young lad was dying from injuries from a road traffic accident. He was a registered organ donor, but his family were not aware of it. Because of the mental trauma of losing a young child, the family decided not to go ahead with organ donation. Affected by this, I remember going home that night and letting my husband Brion know that I wished for him to donate my organs, if that situation ever arose for him to make that decision. That it was just right that my functioning and viable organs were donated to someone who needed it to survive. And that it would be such a waste of a precious organ if it were to be buried or cremated with the person, when it could be the gift of life to another fellow human being. My husband, to whom the topic was a completely alien one, declined to commit to donate his organs at the time, which I respected, and we did not discuss it further then.

Then in the beginning of 2014, one of our best friends, Biju, got diagnosed with myeloma and after chemotherapy and radiation, he would need a stem cell donation to have some hope for a full recovery to be able to enjoy a good quality of life with his young family. All his family & friends including me & Brion, registered as stem cell and organ donors and started supporting one of our friends, Dr. Agimol Pradeep, who is an organ donation specialist nurse, in running campaigns to raise awareness about the topic and register potential stem cell & organ donors among the South Asian population. Brion helped Agimol in a few of these campaigns. Unfortunately, our Biju, did not make it after the stem cell donation and succumbed to complications of low immune status & sepsis.

Exactly 41 days after Biju's passing, Brion had a massive sub arachnoid (brain) haemorrhage and was critically ill. On the 3rd day in intensive care unit, the ICU Consultants, did the Brain stem test and concluded that his brain was not viable. When they informed me of this, I was very upset but found myself saying that he is a registered organ donor and that they could please let the organ donation team know to start preparing Brion for it, as per his wishes. Later that day, Agimol informed me that during one of their previous campaigning sessions, Brion had told the group that if he was ever in this situation, all his organs could be 'taken' as he would not need them, for him to go to heaven. I was so relieved that Agimol had shared this with me at that time and believed that Brion was guiding me through that difficult time in spirit.

He was being prepared for his 2 kidneys, liver and heart to be harvested for donation, but due to complications with the potential recipient and/or some pressure monitoring within his heart, his heart could not be transplanted. He was taken to the operating room on 20th November 2014 for donating his organs. The beautiful thought that some of his organs were still 'alive' in another human being somewhere and were giving them another chance at a new life was extremely reassuring to me in my grief. His kidneys were 'given' to two people in their 40s with young families and the liver went to a young man in his late teenage years. I had received a card from the recipients thanking me for making a difference in their life.

Organ donation as a topic is not something we are exposed to normally. It hits us hard when someone we know is desperate for a new lease of life. My personal inspiration comes from the thought that if I ever needed an organ donation, I would happily go on the waiting list, how then can I hesitate to register as a donor? We should try to reflect on this and ask ourselves where we stand on supporting organ donation and have conversations about this with our loved ones, so they will not be put on the spot when the time arrives but will only be honouring our wishes with the 'gift of life'. The more we talk about it, the less alien the topic becomes and the easier it is for family members to make that decision, at the most difficult time in their lives, especially considering the fact that the decision is irrevocable.

Asian Omelette Recipe

Ingredients:
- 3 Eggs
- 1 Chopped Tomato
- 1 Medium Diced Onion
- 3 Cloves Crushed Garlic
- A Stick Of Ginger
- 1 Red Paprika
- Fresh Coriander Chopped

Spices:
- Garam Masala
- Turmeric (Haldi)
- Haldi
- Salt
- Paprika
- Pepper
- Ghee Butter

(Add chilli powder if you want it extra hot or just leave out)
Serve with: Basmati Rice, Yoghurt and Naan.

Method:

Add ghee butter to a non-stick frying pan, fry onions until golden brown. Add 2 cloves of crushed garlic and 2 teaspoons of ginger and coriander. Add all spices. Add 1.5 teaspoons of each spice. 1/2 teaspoon of salt. Add chopped paprika.

Remove from pan to a bowl. Add 3 eggs to the bowl and stir with the onions and garlic and ginger and paprika. Add oil to the frying pan. Put on a low heat. Add the mixture to the frying pan and cook on a low heat for 10 mins checking the omelette is not sticking.

Side serving: Mix or sprinkle pepper or garam masala to yoghurt for side serving, or grated cucumber/mint sauce to yoghurt. Naan bread if desired.

Pakistani Chicken Recipe

Ingredients:
- 1 Chopped Tomato
- Tomato Puree
- 3 Cloves Crushed Garlic
- A Stick Of Ginger
- Olive Oil
- 1 Medium Diced Onion
- Bio Yoghurt
- Fresh Coriander Chopped
- Chicken Legs or Breasts

Spices:
- Garam Masala
- Turmeric (Haldi)
- Haldi
- Salt
- Paprika
- Pepper

1 Pot For Rice
1 Pot For Chicken

(Add chilli powder if you want it extra hot or just leave out)
Serve with: Basmati Rice, Yoghurt and Naan.

Method:

Add olive oil to pan, fry onions until golden brown. Add 2 cloves of crushed garlic and about ginger Add all spices 1.5 teaspoons of each spice. 1/2 tea spoon of salt. Add more ghee or butter to prevent spices and onions sticking to the pan.

Wash chicken and add to pot with water just slightly underneath the chicken. Add chopped tomatoes and tomato puree, add more water. Up to 1 cup for more sauce, and less than 1 cup for less sauce. Cook for 30 mins on medium heat stirring to reduce water. At the end, add chopped coriander and a tablespoon of garam masala before serving.

Mix or sprinkle pepper or garam masala to yoghurt for side serving or grated cucumber/mint sauce to yoghurt. Cook rice. 2 cups of water to 1 cup of rice. When cooked, add small pieces of butter on top so it melts on top. Sprinkle with water before grilling Naan bread.

Watch online at: **https://bit.ly/3TpcOBt**

Thanks to the Sponsor Anita Myers

GET REAQUAINTED WITH LOVE AND ITS POWER.

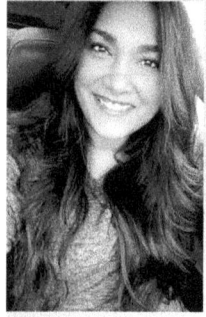

Anita Myers

END EMOTIONAL CHAOS
Life & Relationship Coach
INNERSCOPE365.COM

Emotional Stability Education, Training and Coaching Services

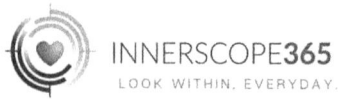

There's more to love...

INNERSCOPE**365**
LOOK WITHIN, EVERYDAY.

Thanks to the Sponsor Hilary Rose

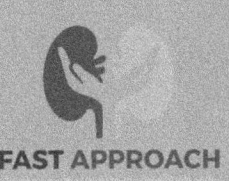

FAST APPROACH

DESTINATION CONCIERGE FOR PEOPLE WITH CHRONIC ILLNESS & DISABILITIES

WHO WE ARE?

"Showing you how to live your best life"
An evolving and inspired company that supports people with Chronic Illnesses & Disabilities to book their ideal holiday so they can create dreams and memories.

WHAT WE DO?

You choose your destination and we will do the rest. Arrange transportation, book your hotel, and organize your excursions. Giving you complete peace of mind, and building on your confidence with small steps of action to improve your health and well-being.

CALL US FOR MORE INFO

 07956 938290

 SERVICES

Public Speaking |Networking |VIP Calls

 MEMBERSHIP

The membership program is dedicated to persons with Chronic Illnesses & Disabilities to receive the most immense support and encouragement to get their lives back on track.

 HOLIDAY CONSULTANTCY

We get to know your likes and dislikes and create a bespoke itinerary that represents you.

 hello@hilaryrose@co.uk
www.hilaryrose.co.uk

Donating Percentage of Proceeds to an Organisation or Charity

For every purchase of this memoir a small donation of money or books will be made to an organisation or charity working on improving patients' lives who are waiting for an organ donation.

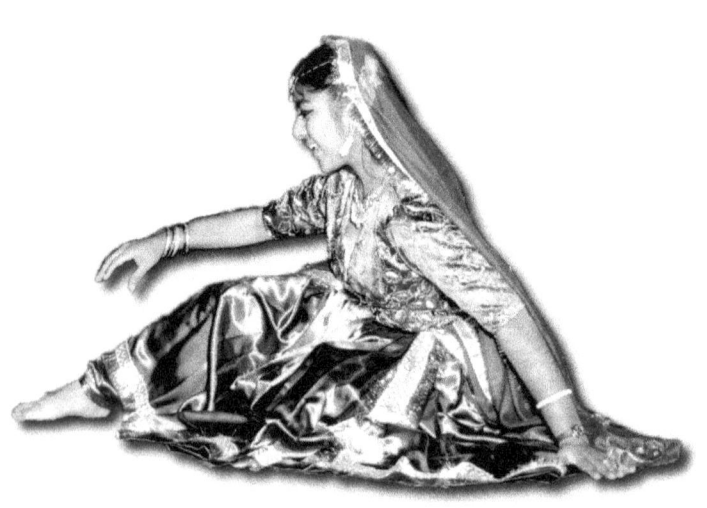

www.ingramcontent.com/pod-product-compliance
Ingram Content Group UK Ltd.
Pitfield, Milton Keynes, MK11 3LW, UK
UKHW012029150625
459729UK00002B/19